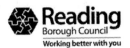

COOKING
FOR FITNESS

PRODUCTION

EDITOR Margaret Nicholls. **CREATIVE DIRECTOR** Gino Tambini.
EDITOR-AT-LARGE Jonathan Haskell. **FOOD PHOTOGRAPHER** Clive Bozzard-Hill.
FOOD STYLIST Liz O'Keefe. **FOOD ASSISTANT** Helen Rance.
FOOD ASSISTANT Hannah Searle. **FILMING CO-ORDINATOR** Hannah Mitchell.
NUTRITIONIST Fiona Hunter. **COVER & PORTRAIT PHOTOGRAPHER** Neil Cooper.

PRINTED BY OLUŞUR

HASKELL
PUBLISHING

First published 2019 by Haskell Publishing, a division of James Haskell Health & Fitness Ltd
www.jameshaskell.com

ISBN 9780995544642

Member 2018
ipg
Independent Publishers Guild

FSC
www.fsc.org
MIX
Paper from
responsible sources
FSC™ C140853

Sebastian's Action Trust

A percentage of the proceeds from the sale of this book
will be donated to Sebastian's Action Trust, of which
James is one of the patrons. Charity number: 1151146

JAMES HASKELL HEALTH & FITNESS HELPS YOU ACHIEVE A HEALTHIER AND FITTER LIFESTYLE

We do this by delivering professional fitness and nutrition advice in a simple, clear and easy-to-understand format. In conjunction with the development of our own range of clean and certified sports supplements, this allows the individual to achieve the lifestyle balance that is right for them. All of our supplements, training and cook books are exclusively created and designed in Britain. JHHF is proud to support and work with British talent, in order to fully utilise the great skill-set this country boasts.

MADE IN BRITAIN

COOKING
FOR FITNESS

JAMES HASKELL
& OMAR MEZIANE

ALSO BY JAMES HASKELL

**INTRODUCTION TO BECOMING
AND REMAINING RUGBYFIT**
ISBN: 97812526202130

PERFECT FIT
ISBN: 9781473648739

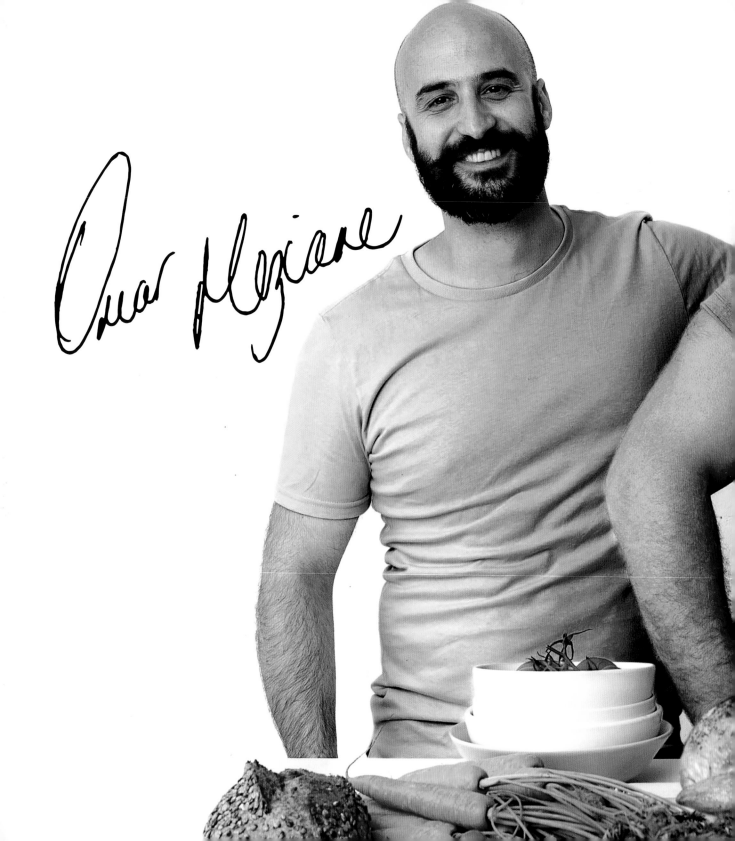

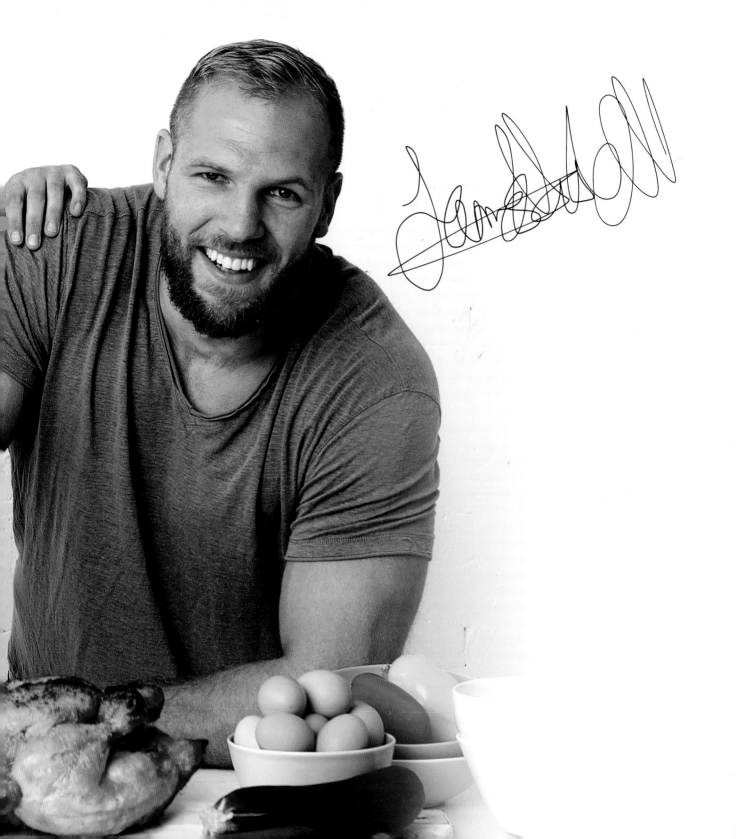

CONTENTS

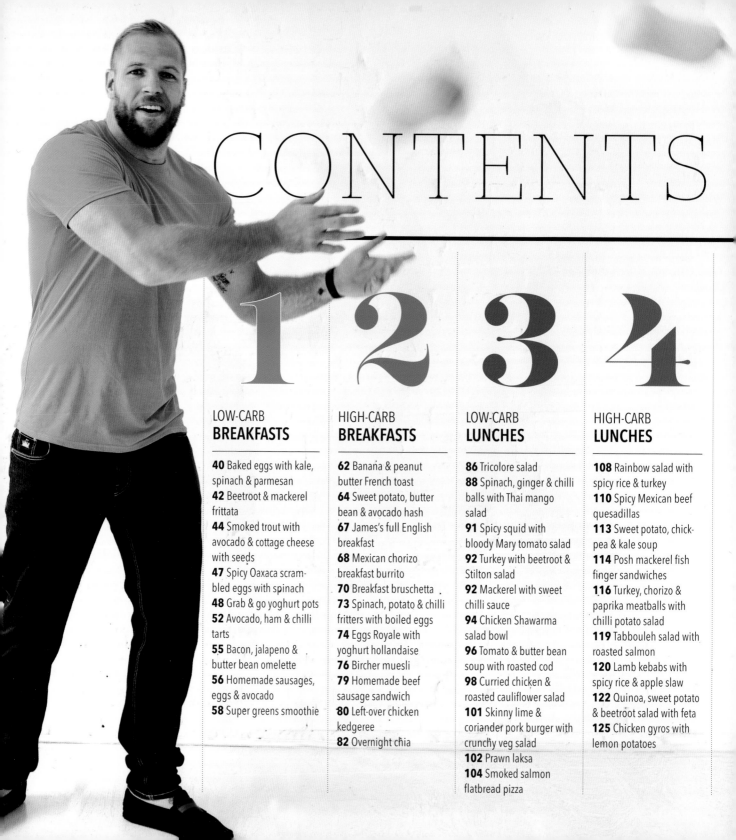

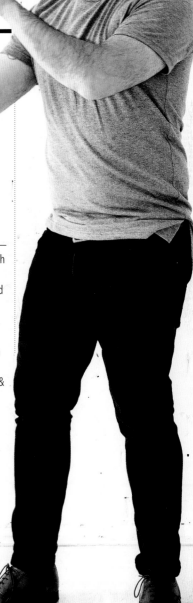

5

LOW-CARB
DINNERS

6

HIGH-CARB
DINNERS

7

PRE-TRAINING
SNACKS

8

POST-TRAINING
SNACKS

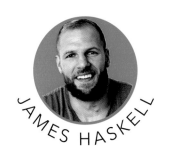

WELCOME TO
COOKING FOR FITNESS

It's been a couple of years since I wrote my first training guide, *Introduction to Becoming and Remaining Rugby Fit*, and now I'm extremely excited to welcome you to my latest book, *Cooking For Fitness.*

The idea behind this book is to provide you with healthy recipes that will keep you in shape throughout your rugby season or, if you don't play rugby, recipes that will teach you how to eat smart to fuel your general training.

Throughout my 15 years as a sportsman, I have played around the world in countries such as France, Japan, and New Zealand, and been lucky enough to work with some of the best coaches, nutritionists and fitness trainers out there.

However, budding rugby players are not my only focus. I hope that anyone wanting to get into shape finds value in the pages of my guides.

My objective is always to write in-depth books that will help you achieve your goals – whether they're focused on rugby, fitness, aesthetics or general health.

Rugby Fit was step one. *Lean Gains* was my second release, which focused more on muscle-building. Most recently, my body transformation book *Perfect Fit* explained how to lose weight and/or gain muscle in the most comprehensive way, covering everything you need to know, from beginners to advanced.

Perfect Fit details how to train both at home and in the gym, and explains how to build a nutrition plan that works for life, not just for short-term results. If you missed it, you can still find it in most book stores or online.

> *If you want to perform well, you need to fuel your body in the right way*

With *Cooking for Fitness*, I have come back to my rugby roots and teamed up with my favourite chef, Omar Meziane, to create super-healthy, incredibly tasty recipes that are great for rugby players and anyone serious about eating in the right way. If you are a fan of my website www.jameshaskell.com or my YouTube channel www.youtube.com/thejameshaskell, you will have seen me cooking up a storm with Omar on many occasions.

He has been the Wasps Rugby team chef, as well as cooking for the GB Rowing team, and is currently executive chef for the England Men's Football team. Like me, Omar understands that eating healthily can be difficult and requires commitment, but that it does not have to be boring.

Everything I have ever written or talked about in regards to health and fitness always expresses the importance of nutrition. It really is the key.

If you want to perform on the rugby field or in the gym, you need to fuel your body in the right way. If you are casual about your nutrition, you will become a casualty of it.

Cooking for Fitness has you covered from breakfast to dinner. We talk you through pre- and post-workout snacks as well as high- and low-carb meals.

This book is about helping you to perform in your chosen sport and/or helping you to build muscle. Whatever your goal is, you will be able to find a recipe that caters to your needs. You will also be able to adapt these recipes to fit your exact nutritional needs and preferences.

When Omar and I were writing this, we were committed to creating fast, tasty and easy-to-make meals.

You will see that we have gone for good, wholesome foods and not tried to make anything overly complicated. You don't need to be buying expensive superfoods or weird and wonderful health products.

Some of our recipes are high in calories, some even include refined carbs, but if you train properly for your sport and work hard, all of this will fit nicely into your diet.

Many of the recipes in *Cooking for Fitness* will take you no more than 20 minutes to prepare. If any do require longer, simply cook double, triple or quadruple what you need and save the meals for later in the week. Alternatively, use a day off to prep your meals for the week ahead. I do this all the time and it's extremely helpful with my schedule.

I hope you enjoy eating these meals as much as Omar and I enjoyed creating them.

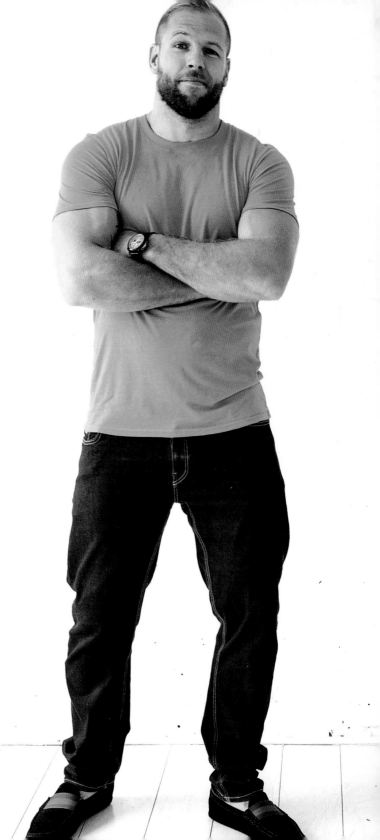

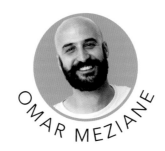

MEET THE CHEF: OMAR MEZIANE

For me it all started back at the Wasps training ground in Acton. Feeding elite rugby players was a challenge and, at first, I didn't succeed. In my mind, cooking for athletes entailed steaming everything in sight and never using any salt or sugar.

As you can probably imagine, when an entire squad of rugby players are unimpressed with the food they are being offered, they can be very vocal about it.

I knew I had to go back to the drawing board.

I began to cook food that I loved and food that excited me. It was an instant success and gave me the confidence to carry it further. My style of food is very loosely based around my heritage, with lots of Mediterranean influences and plenty of herbs and spices.

James would wander into the kitchen at Wasps most afternoons. We would always talk food and about how he could cook better meals for himself at home. It's those numerous conversations that inspired the recipes in this book.

We wanted to create a collection of delicious dishes with ingredients that can be found in any supermarket. You will not find any of them calling for bio-dynamic honey or mushrooms that have been harvested only when Mercury is in transit.

I am lucky enough to work with some of the world's finest performance nutritionists on a daily basis. This relationship is symbiotic and I rely on their knowledge of both the science and the individual athlete. Together we tailor menus to their particular needs. The tricky part is making the food tasty.

Over the years I have been working in professional sport – from Wasps to GB Rowing team to the England Men's Football team – I have developed quite a repertoire of recipes.

The recipes in this book are all based around these years of experience working with the world's finest sports men and women and, of course, the big man James Haskell.

The recipes are great as they are, but do feel free to change the protein source or mix and match the carbs. To make it easier, we have divided them into low-carb and high-carb chapters. However, as James explains, you can adapt the dishes according to the calories or macronutrients you need, whether you're eating for muscle gain, fat loss, to improve your performance or purely to stay fit and fuel your training.

But remember that great food starts with great ingredients. Don't be tempted to cut corners and buy a pot of pre-wilted spinach or a pre-roasted chicken. The fun is in cooking and the satisfaction is in eating what you have prepared.

For athletes, food is important on so many levels. It needs to support them nutritionally and enable them to perform and recover. But first and foremost, I believe that food should be delicious. And that eating a balanced, colourful and delicious diet will only benefit you.

Happy cooking,

> *We wanted to create recipes with ingredients that can be found in any supermarket*

Omar Meziane

OMAR AND ME

You may have picked up this book because you have some understanding of who I am, who Omar is, or simply because you like the look of the food. If the latter is true and you have no idea who I am or what I do, allow me to explain...

My name is James Haskell and I am a professional rugby player for Northampton Saints and, when selected, England. I played over 200 times for Wasps and have played 75 times for England so far. Over the course of my career, I have been fortunate enough to play all over the world and work with some quality nutritionists and chefs.

My life has been about eating (and eating well) for as long as I can remember. Food is a very important part of my daily routine and over the years I have learnt how to prepare and eat food that is both healthy and tasty.

Chefs like Omar have shown me how to take good sources of protein, carbohydrates and fat, and make delicious meals that hit my daily nutritional requirements.

Omar especially has shown me that you can eat well but still have all the flavour you get from not-so-healthy foods.

I don't want to bang on about eating "clean" as everyone gets their knickers in a twist about it. What I personally mean by "clean" food is food that is free from additives and preservatives. Trans fats, refined sugars, sweeteners, flavourings and high-sodium foods tend to be the ones to avoid.

Everything I preach in the pages of *Cooking for Fitness*, I practise.

At the time of writing this I had to overhaul my entire diet for the new rugby season, before which I enjoyed five weeks off. This was very much needed, but the fact is that eating and drinking whatever you want comes at a price. The penalty is weight gain, and all of it in the form of body fat.

I needed to reduce my weight and body fat percentage, otherwise I'd be running around the field like a milk float with a low battery.

I approached this by eating well, tracking my calories and macros and training very hard. All of these steps are laid out for you in this book.

If you want to know more about me and/or my rugby life then head over to www.jameshaskell.com or follow me on social media. I am constantly uploading behind-the-scenes content and sharing fitness tips.

🐦 @JamesHaskell

📷 @JamesHask

▶ www.youtube.com/thejameshaskell

f www.facebook.com/JameshaskellJHHF

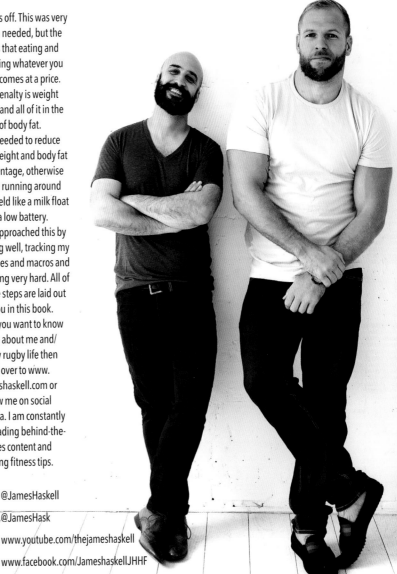

THE IMPORTANCE OF NUTRITION

Let me be clear right now, I am not a qualified nutritionist, nor am I a registered dietitian.

However, throughout my rugby career I've been lucky enough to work with some of the UK's top sports nutrition experts, including performance nutritionist Matt Lovell, strength and conditioning expert Phil Learney and Dr Graeme Close, who is senior lecturer in sports nutrition at Liverpool John Moores University.

The main lesson I've learned from them is that the basics are all you need to succeed. And the basic rules of nutrition have not changed. Simply put, it comes down to calories in vs calories out.

CRAZY DIETS

Remember that eating badly or trying stupid fad diets will only cause more problems in the long run.

You're likely to get short-term results from most extreme dietary methods (juicing, Atkins, etc), but trust me, you will pay the price down the line.

If you starve your body and later decide that, actually, you quite like food and probably need it to function, you will put the weight back on just as quickly as you lost it. On top of the return weight gain, you will find that your body fat percentage (those wobbly bits) has actually increased.

Fat loss teas or pills, or lemon-juice and cayenne-pepper shakes are not the answer. Instead of all this craziness, why don't you try something that is sustainable, worthwhile and that won't damage your health?

Cooking for Fitness will shine an accurate light on how the right approach to food can help you to progress your fitness, nutritional and healthy lifestyle goals.

BEING SENSIBLE

If you want to perform to the best of your ability, then you simply have to eat well. You will never become the rugby player or athlete you want to be if you don't eat the right foods at the right times. Even if you can't think of anything worse than playing rugby, and all you want is to be happy in your own skin, diet is the key to achieving the results you want. You need to fuel your body with the right amount of calories to perform and recover, while maintaining your ideal body composition.

I am going to give you a quick overview of what you need to: a) use this book properly and b) guide your nutrition choices.

If you like what you read here, then you can build a much more specific and subjective diet plan by reading *Perfect Fit*.

GETTING STARTED

Whatever your goal may be, the best way to get started is to assess how you're eating now and what you're putting into your body over the course of a typical week so you can understand what your daily average calorie intake is. Once you understand how you actually eat, you will have a number that you can then tweak here and there, or implement a total dietary overhaul.

The first time I did this I was shocked by how little protein I was consuming and by the amount of fats and sugars hidden inside what I was eating.

I always thought I was eating really well, but it turned out I needed to improve things *a lot*.

MY FITNESS PAL

I track my daily dietary intake using the smart phone app MyFitnessPal. I am sure there are other apps out there, but MFP is the one that I find works best for my needs.

The app is extremely easy to use. You simply input what you are eating throughout the day. For example, for breakfast you could log one sachet of oats, a tablespoon of nut butter and a banana. You can also scan in the barcodes of most products.

With every recipe in this book we have included a barcode that links to the MFP app, so you can instantly track your calories and your macros.

If an app feels a bit OTT for you personally, you can track your progress in any way you like. Food diaries are a great method, too. Just keep in mind that apps such as MFP will give you very accurate calculations of calories and macros.

BASIC NUTRITION

Understanding how food fuels your body will help you choose the right recipes at the right times.

We all need calories in order to survive, and they should come from the three macronutrients:

1. Protein (repairs torn tissue, encouraging muscle recovery and growth)
2. Carbohydrates (provide energy and muscular strength)
3. Fat (provides energy and protects vital organs)

These three macros are what your body needs in order to achieve optimum health and physical function. Your daily calorie count and amount of macros should be goal dependent.

For example, building muscle requires a high-calorie, high-protein, high-carbohydrate diet. Fats do need to play a role, but very much a minor role when muscle-building is your goal.

Whatever anyone tells you, if you want to build muscle you need to be in a calorie surplus, ie, consume more calories than you burn, through daily life and through your training.

In the case of fat loss, which we will look into in more detail later, simply put, you need to be in a calorie deficit.

I know there are a lot of horror stories about carbohydrates out there, but the fact of the matter is that you cannot train hard consistently or build muscle without eating carbs.

While this book may be more for sportsmen and women and those who train hard, I still want to explain how it can work for fat loss goals. If you are clever about it, you can adapt all of these recipes to your own personal goals and achieve the aesthetic results you're after.

Weight loss, fat loss, any kind of whittling down is simply about calories. Energy (calories) from food and drink vs energy (calories) out through exercise and activity is how you will change your body. Once you understand this, you can start to think about what role the three macronutrients will play within your calorie count.

If you train and your goal is to lose weight or fat, your carbohydrates (such as oats, rice, potato, fruit etc) should be consumed pre- and post-training only. The rest of the time, you should be focusing on protein, fats and non-starchy vegetables (such as leaves, broccoli, cauliflower, courgettes, asparagus, onions, green beans etc).

I strongly recommend that you take any recipe you like the look of and adapt it to your own specific goals. While some books specialise in fat loss, muscle gain or overall health goals, I wanted to write something that can be tailored to the individual.

Whatever your age or aim, this book can help, once you understand the nutrition basics.

MORE ON MACROS

As I've mentioned in the previous pages, there are three macronutrients that should make up your overall daily calorie count: protein, carbohydrates and fat. Here is a little more detail about the role they play in your diet.

1. PROTEIN

Meat, poultry, fish, egg whites, dairy, beans, pulses, nuts, seeds, soy products, protein powders, mycoproteins such as Quorn, etc.

Protein creates, maintains and repairs tissues inside the body. Our bodies already make non-essential-amino-acids, but we need to get our essential amino acids from external food sources such as meat, chicken and fish. Hence why these amino acids are called essential – because we don't make them naturally.

Vegans and vegetarians need to eat a variety of proteins during the day in order to get their essential amino acids. You'd be surprised by how many tell me that they get all the protein they need from a plate of broccoli!

Combinations such as rice and beans, nuts and grains, or even produce such as quinoa, will help non-meat-eaters out with their essential amino acid intake. Unfortunately, these foods will see their starchy carbohydrate numbers skyrocket, so they may need to keep an eye on this.

SUPPLEMENTS

Protein powders are also a source of essential amino acids; however, they should not be your only or even frequent source. Supplements are exactly that – supplements to your diet – and protein shakes are not going to make you massive.

Your body needs to digest proper food. Protein powders should only play a role once you have the basics of your nutrition nailed down and are looking for something to make your macro requirements a little easier.

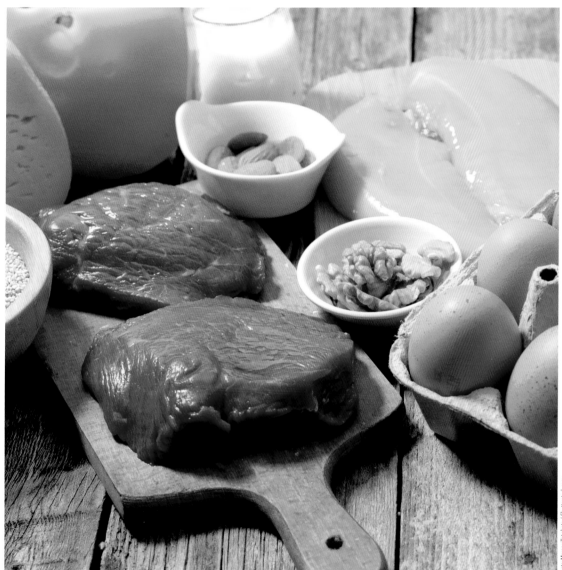

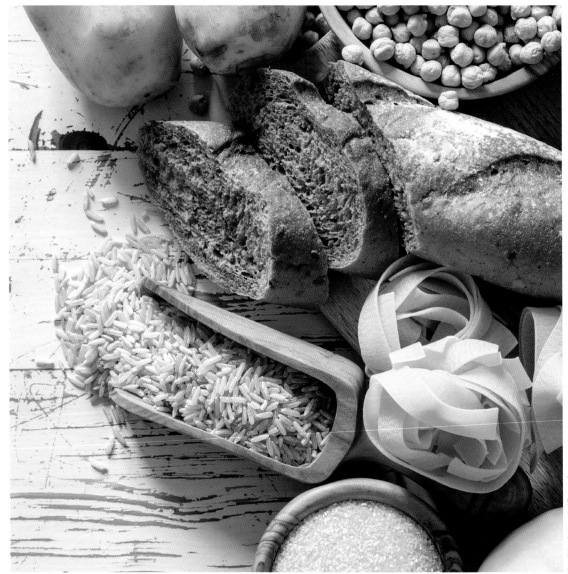

2. CARBOHYDRATES

Oats, wholegrains, rice, potato, fruit, bread, pasta, cereals, beans and pulses, etc.

Carbohydrates are your body's absolute favourite source of energy.

As I have already mentioned, carbohydrates have replaced fats as the bad guys in recent years. Neither of these is true.

Let me be very clear, no food is going to make you 'fat'. Proteins, fats and carbs should all be consumed as part of a healthy diet. Calories and timing of food intake are what should be manipulated.

Not only does Sedentary Sally need carbs in her diet, Active Andy (excuse the cheese) isn't going to be active for very long if he decides carbs make him fat. Active Andy will probably have to retire, to be honest.

The fact is, if you do any form of physical activity and especially if you are a performance athlete, carbs need to play a starring role in your diet.

If you are trying to train or play sport every week and are eating like a *MensHealth* cover model in ketosis, you are going to put yourself at risk of injury and fatigue.

Once again, eating carbs will not make you fat; eating more than your body requires will make you fat. Your level of activity has to match your diet. Remember this lesson and you will never stray too far out of shape.

> *Complex carbs are essential for fuelling training and enhancing performance*

There are in fact different types of carbs that work differently inside the body. Simple carbs such as refined sugars and fruit are used very quickly and give immediate energy. Complex carbs such as oats, potatoes and wholegrain cereals give a more prolonged energy release.

The main carbohydrate we want to focus on in this book is the complex variety, as for performance athletes, complex carbs are essential for fuelling training, aiding recovery and enhancing performance.

If your goal is muscle gain then again complex carbs will need to be eaten at every meal.

You can be more relaxed about simple carbs pre- and post-workout.

The body uses glucose as an immediate energy source, so if ingested pre-training, it will be put straight to good use.

Post-workout, simple sugars induce an insulin spike. Insulin then helps transport nutrients to your muscles quickly, encouraging rebuild. That is why some of the recipes in *Cooking for Fitness* have sugar and refined carbs in them. These are for post-training.

Complex carbs are the only carbs to eat if your goal is fat loss. Eat these types of carbs pre- and post-training only.

3. FAT

Nuts, nut butters, whole eggs, avocados, oils, oily fish, fatty meats, etc.

Fats are your body's secondary energy source. They also protect vital organs, allow your body to absorb vitamins A, D and E, and they regulate hormones.

The human body cannot function without fats, yet for many years they have been demonised by the media.

Both saturated and unsaturated fats should play a role in your daily diet and neither should be avoided.

Saturated fats come from sources such as meat and dairy. They should play a small, but ever-present role in your daily diet.

Unsaturated fats (which divide into two sub-categories: polyunsaturated and monounsaturated) come from sources such as nuts and oily fish and contain essential fatty acids. Much like essential amino acids, EFAs are not made within the body naturally and therefore must be ingested via your diet.

MICRONUTRIENTS

There are two broad categories of micronutrient: vitamins and minerals. Think of your micronutrients as the keys to your macronutrients.

Although micros have negligible calorific value, they are essential for hormonal health, metabolism, immune support and organ function.

Fruit and vegetables and other plant-based foods are a great source of micros, which is why you should never neglect your greens, kids!

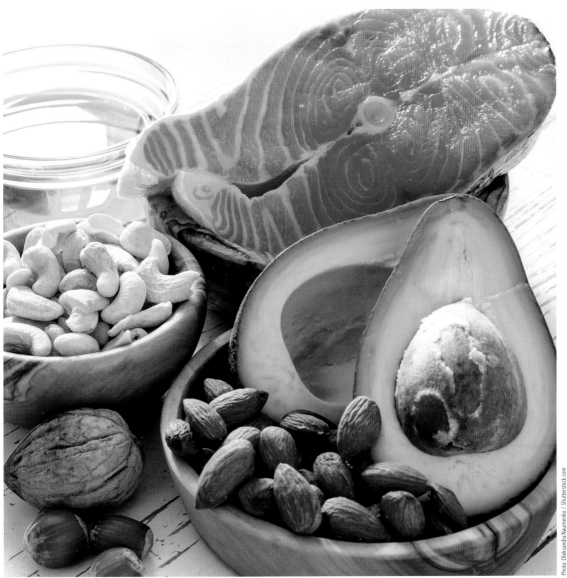

Photo: Oleksandra Naumenko / Shutterstock.com

HOW TO USE THIS BOOK

You will see from the recipes in *Cooking for Fitness* that we have you covered for breakfast, lunch, dinner, snacks and shakes.

We have given full nutritional breakdowns for every recipe so that you can see the exact amounts of calories, protein, carbohydrates and fat contained in each one. This will make it easy for you to create your own eating plan according to your goals.

And alongside this nutritional information, every recipe in this book has a barcode you can scan directly into the MyFitnessPal app. Turn to page 196 for more information about how the app works.

In addition, all of the recipes can be edited to fit your own specific dietary/training/aesthetic needs. The reason we haven't made everything super rigid is because everybody has a different goal and, truthfully, when it comes to nutrition, there are pros and cons to everything.

With performance goals and/or muscular gains in mind, you don't have to be nearly as rigid as you would if you were 100 per cent focused on fat loss.

Omar and I want to give you guys the freedom to add and remove ingredients to suit you. For example, the Banana bread recipe, page 190, contains sugar. This is ideal for pre- or post-training, but not ideal if you want to really lean down. So we have given you the option to replace the sugar with a sweetener like stevia (eg, Truvia). In the Homemade beef sausage sandwich, page 79, you may want to swap the white bread for a lower-carb version.

Performance sport nutrition requires a different strategy to 'normal' eating habits

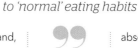

If you are tracking your macros as I have suggested, the MyFitnessPal app will make these decisions for you. For example, if you have exceeded your carbs for the day, then remove the carbohydrates from the recipe you fancy.

Another way we have set up the book for ease of use is by splitting the recipes into low-carbohydrate and high-carbohydrate chapters.

The meals that are low in carbohydrates are made up of mostly proteins and fats.

Just a quick note here that all vegetables, even non-starchy veg (eg, broccoli) and other things that you may not expect (eg, whey protein), do contain carbohydrates.

While you will not, in the main, be eating starchy/complex carbs (eg, potatoes and rice) during low-carb meals, there will be some carbohydrate grams picked up here and there. This is absolutely not a problem. I am simply noting it in case you are tracking on MyFitnessPal and see grams of carbs where you expected there to be none. These carbs are incidentals and not to be worried about.

If you train a lot, or are a performance athlete who prioritises recovery, then eating carbs on your day off will not be an issue.

HOW TO TAILOR THIS BOOK FOR YOU
Please remember as you read through this book that I am speaking to a multitude of people with a multitude of goals and needs. For example, some of you may be super active; others not so much. In short, you will all require different amounts of nutrients to power you throughout your day.

To bring things back to their most basic form, whatever your goal is, it comes down to calories in vs calories out. If you want to gain you have to be in a surplus; if you want to lose you have to be in a deficit; and if you want performance you need consistency and the right balance of macros.

PERFORMANCE SPORT

Performance sport nutrition requires a different strategy to 'normal' eating habits. On the whole, things like intermittent fasting – or fasting that affects the amount of calories you eat in a day – is not going to work for you. The same goes for aggressive carb cycling. These are great tools, but not for performance athletes, or certainly not for those in season.

Not only do you have to fuel your daily training, you have to aid your physical recovery, work towards your overall body composition goals and perform at 100 per cent.

More than anything, you need to get the balance right between your calorie, protein, carbohydrate and fat intake.

If you don't fuel your body properly you will feel tired, lose focus and potentially under-perform. If you feel good in a match but your energy fades, this could be a sign you're not eating well enough.

You will need to put some time into perfecting this. Experiment by trying out different meals before normal training sessions.

If you eat too much or not enough and have any negative reactions, it's obviously better to find this out in a training session instead of during a huge game.

This is the same if you are going to try taking supplements, such as pre-workouts or caffeine. Remember that everyone reacts differently.

MUSCLE GAIN

For muscle gain you will need to fuel your training but also eat a calorie surplus to promote muscle growth. This calorie surplus should come predominantly from proteins and carbohydrates.

In my experience, men tend to think that they can instantly gain muscle and women fear that they will pick up a dumbbell and immediately puff up like Arnold Schwarzenegger. Neither will happen. Your body takes time to adapt to any changes you are trying to implement. Trust me.

FAT LOSS

The main focus of this book is performance and muscle gain. However, it can also work for weight loss and/or fat loss. To get leaner, you need to be in a calorie deficit, and your calories need to be made up predominantly of lean protein, healthy fats and non-starchy vegetable sources. Restrict the starchy carbohydrates to pre- and post-training. You have fat as your alternative energy macro in every other meal.

Once you begin tracking your daily intake you can start taking away or adding to your calories and macros to achieve your desired goals.

Whatever that goal is, be patient and remember that results take time!

EATING TOWARDS YOUR GOALS

Now you know what foods your body needs, it's time to figure out how to manipulate them to achieve your goals. **We have all heard fitness "gurus" say that you can't achieve any results at all without the right diet, but the fact of the matter is, you can't achieve any transformation at all if you aren't doing the right training either.**

The two go hand in hand. If one is not right then you won't progress. You need to train and you need to work hard.

This book is not a training guide and I am not trying to make it one, but this book will only help you if you have the right work ethic when it comes to training. If you need guidance, my last book, *Perfect Fit,* has full eight-week and 12-week training guides for both fat loss and muscle gain.

One thing you will notice in *Cooking for Fitness* is that I have not been specific about the amount of food you should be eating at meal times or throughout the day. The reason behind this is simply that everyone is different and that each reader has a different goal in mind.

You can double quantities and remove items from the recipes as you see fit

Portion sizes, calories and macros depend on your own desired outcomes. As discussed on page 12, tracking your food will help you figure out your own personal numbers. While there are guideline amounts in the recipes, you can double quantities or remove items as you see fit.

HOW MANY MEALS SHOULD I EAT IN A DAY?

Not so long ago the advice was to eat small, frequent meals throughout the day in order to boost metabolism. FORGET THIS IMMEDIATELY.

Eating six meals a day is no better than eating five. Having three meals and two snacks is no better than having four solid meals.

When good dietitians, nutritionists and coaches instruct you to split up your meals and snacks throughout the day, it will be because of the following factors...

1. The quantities you personally need to eat on a daily basis. For example, trying to get 3000 calories (of clean food – large pizzas don't apply) into three meals will be hard. But if you spread your daily intake across five or six meals, you're going to feel better throughout the day (as in not over- or under-full) and you will hit your numbers with ease.

2. There are optimal times to eat during the day. For example, pre- and post-training meals and snacks are going to ensure that you get the best out of your session in terms of energy release, results and recovery.

EATING AS A RUGBY PLAYER/ATHLETE

As a rugby player, I eat to fuel my training and keep my body in shape. This means that I need to get the balance of my macros right. I have carbs, protein and fats in every meal throughout the day, albeit in the right quantities.

Without going into my specific numbers (as they do not apply to you), my macro split is 40% protein, 40% carbohydrates and 20% fats.

I am constantly thinking about two things: fuelling my training so I perform well, and recovering from my training so I continue to perform well. I do not carb load. Ever. I used to do this, but I find that keeping things constant throughout the week works best for me.

I train twice a day, one on-field session, the other off-field.

On the right is an example of what I eat on a typical day – I am not going to put amounts next to foods as I don't want you to copy what I do. You are not me and you personally may need less or more. Remember that I am a 120kg forward who wants to maintain size, performance and certain body fat levels without having to do lots of weights. So diet is massive for me. I am constantly tracking, tweaking and adding to what I do.

You will know what your own body composition goals are going to be. Do you need to be big and heavy, but able to last 80 minutes? Or do you need to be lean and quick, and feel confident that you have enough energy to perform?

When you're eating for performance, there is a balance between fuelling your training and trying to stay as lean/big and healthy as possible. That is why tracking your food is essential. You can then tweak things, after assessing how you feel during games, post-training, or depending on your body fat percentage. Throughout my season, the amount of calories I eat changes, I would say, every 12 weeks. Not by much, but by little tweaks.

TRAINING DAY

BREAKFAST
- Eggs
- Chicken sausage
- Toast
- Probiotic drink
- Protein porridge
- 2 litres of water
- Coffee with whole milk

DRIVE TO TRAINING
- Protein shake with carbs and greens supplement en route

POST-1ST TRAINING SESSION
- Chicken or fish
- Brown rice or potato
- Broccoli
- 1 litre of water

POST-2ND TRAINING SESSION
- Sea bass
- Olives
- Sun-dried tomato rice
- 1 litre of water

SNACK
- Banana & almond seedy bars, recipe page 176

DINNER
- Courgette beef lasagne, recipe page 134
- 1 litre of water

GAME DAY

I know I will get questions on how I eat pre-match so here is an example of what I do on match days (usual kick off at 3pm):

BREAKFAST
- Eggs
- Toast
- Porridge with protein powder
- 2 litres of water with electrolytes

PRE-MATCH
- Salmon
- Brown rice or potato
- Broccoli
- Protein pancakes
- 2 litres of water
- 1 espresso

POST-MATCH (IMMEDIATE)
Protein shake with a carb source

POST-MATCH (2 HRS)
- Chicken
- Rice
- Vegetables
- 1 or 2 litres of water

EVENING MEAL
- Pizza (this is my go-to refeed/ cheat after a game)

EATING FOR MUSCLE GAIN

To gain muscle you need to be in a calorie surplus, made up predominantly of protein and carbohydrates.

You will do this by eating more – a lot more. But this is not a green card to pig out on chocolate, crisps and pizza. Extra calories need to be healthy.

Please don't go mad from the start and try to eat huge quantities of food from day one. You will not be able to do it and will probably give up after a few days. You want to gradually increase the amount of food you are eating week on week. Muscle building is progressive and it takes time.

As I said before, protein and carbs will be your best friends on your path to gaining muscle.

EAT ENOUGH FOOD

I get messages all the time from men especially, saying that they are training hard but just can't put on size. While there are hard gainers out there, most people simply aren't eating enough food, or enough of the right food.

It's a common complaint and often when I question them I find out they are eating 2000 calories a day and think it's enough. Trust me, if you have been eating your arse off and have seen no progress, then you just aren't eating enough. There are no ifs or buts. Even if you have a fast metabolism, it just means you have to eat more. You need to track your food to get a calorie figure to work from, which you can then add to, to help you gain size.

Just like burning a large quantity of body fat, gaining size is a full-time job. It takes hard work and commitment and is something you have to wake up thinking about and live throughout the day.

Below, I've given you an example of what I was eating when I was gaining size. Again, I haven't included the amounts because if I do people will wrongly copy them. Numbers are subjective, please remember that.

Hopefully, these examples will help you understand how to eat if you want to build muscle. Skipping breakfast and having a supermarket sandwich for lunch just won't cut it.

MONITOR YOUR PROGRESS

My advice for those wanting to build muscle is to sort your diet out and eat consistently with some added calories for two weeks. I would suggest you make these calorie increases through your protein and carbohydrate intake specifically. Fats rarely need to exceed 1g per kg of body weight,

BREAKFAST
♦ Eggs
♦ Toast
♦ Steak
♦ Nuts
♦ Porridge with protein powder
♦ Probiotic drink
♦ 2 litres of water
♦ 1 coffee

EN-ROUTE TO TRAINING
♦ Protein shake with carb source and greens supplement

POST-TRAINING
♦ Sea bass with ginger & tamari, recipe page 152

♦ Boiled white rice
♦ Edamame beans

AFTERNOON SNACK
♦ Chicken curry and rice
♦ Protein waffles, Greek yoghurt and agave syrup

DINNER
♦ Sirloin steak
♦ 5 per cent fat oven chips
♦ Broccoli mash
♦ 2 litres of water
♦ Yoghurt, nut butter and granola
Sometimes I would throw in a shake before bed at 50 per cent protein, 50 per cent carbs

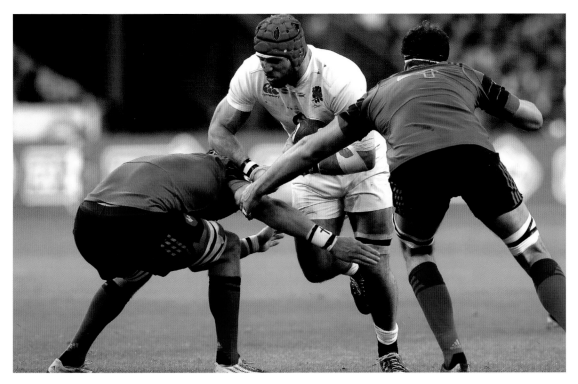

unless following a ketogenic diet. You will then have a full understanding of the amount of food you are eating and aiming to eat to gain. If you don't see any changes, or make any gains, then you need to add to your calories and macros once again.

As a rule, I would add 250 calories a time, when you are looking to increase the amount of food you are eating. If you are already eating 2g of protein to 1kg of body weight, then you would look to make up these new calories from carbohydrates. So you would add to the amount of carbs you are having daily. You do not really want to exceed

2.5g to 1kg of body weight for protein.

You will see changes in your body by tracking your progress through the ways I have suggested on page 30, ie photos and your weight. You then stay at this new calorific amount for another two weeks and see how you go.

Repeat this process until you have gained the amount of size you want.

In my book *Perfect Fit,* I take you through how to build your own personal nutrition plan, including calories and macros. This information will give you lessons for life that you can keep revisiting for your goals.

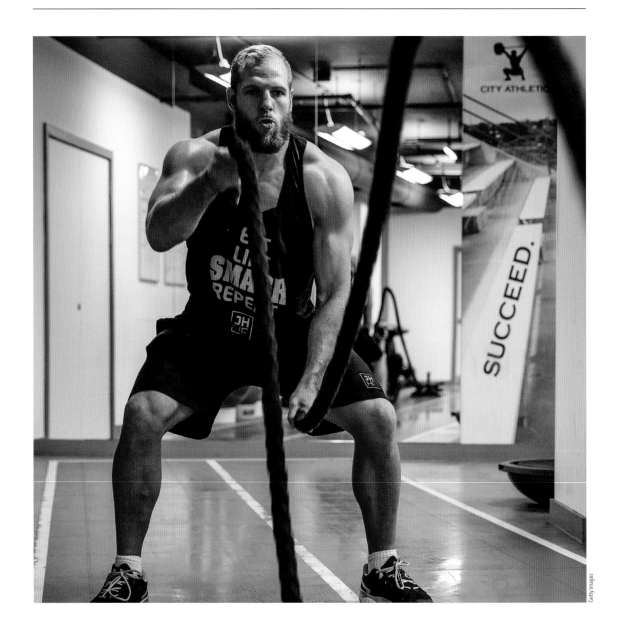

EATING FOR FAT LOSS

While *Cooking for Fitness* is not directly tailored to those seeking fat loss, you can still get real benefits from using this book if fat loss is your goal.

If you have taken on board what I have said about eating in line with your energy demands, you will start transforming your diet and, in turn, change your body.

Following these guidelines will mean that you are eating differently on training days compared with rest days or low activity days.

In basic terms this means on training days you will have carbohydrates pre- and post-training as your fuel. You will then be using fats to power everything else you are doing. On rest days, fats will be your go-to energy macro and you will be leaving complex carbs alone.

On the right is how you would eat for a fat loss goal, using the recipes in this book. If you stick to this structure you will get the results you want.

It's really important to understand that if your goal is fat loss then you need to be eating less than you are eating now. As I have explained, macros are super important, for example what type of carbs you eat and whether you are on a training day or not. Yet in its simplest form fat loss is about reducing your daily calories safely, healthily and slowly so you get results. I go into this in far more detail in my book *Perfect Fit*.

TRAINING DAY
BREAKFAST
♦ Smoked trout with avocado & cottage cheese with seeds, recipe page 44
POST-TRAINING
♦ Rainbow salad with spicy rice & turkey, recipe page 108
AFTERNOON MEAL/SNACK
♦ Omelette and avocado
DINNER
Satay chicken with papaya & chilli salad, recipe page 133

NON-TRAINING DAY
BREAKFAST
♦ Spicy Oaxaca scrambled eggs with spinach, recipe page 47
LUNCH
♦ Curried chicken & roasted cauliflower salad, recipe page 98
AFTERNOON SNACK/MEAL
Protein waffles and Greek yoghurt
DINNER
♦ Curried pork chop with Indian cucumber salad, recipe page 140

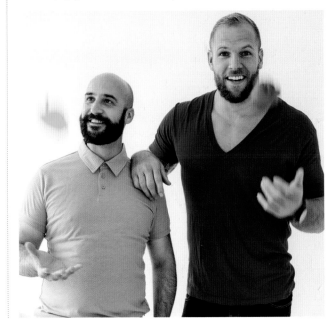

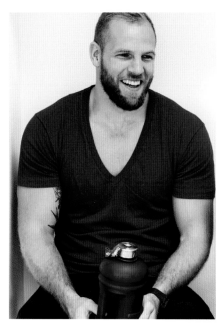

HYDRATION

You will have seen in my personal diet examples that I noted 1 litre of water here or 2 litres of water there. Whatever your goal, hydration will play a huge role.

Water is something that I have neglected in the past, and I paid the price for this in my performance. I now track my daily hydration by using MyFitnessPal.

Staying well hydrated is important for mental and physical reasons. It will aid concentration and effectively allow metabolic function within the body.

If I am dehydrated I feel sluggish and sore, and I notice a significant drop in my cardio performance. Being well-hydrated makes me feel so much better and, more importantly, diminishes the likelihood of muscular injury, illness, headaches and, ultimately, the chances of regression or hindered performances.

Personally, I try to drink between 5 and 6 litres a day. This is a lot and I am sure that some experts out there would suggest less. I would advise between 4 and 5, but it's best to sip it throughout the day as drinking too much water in a short space of time may cause serious medical problems.

One way to check your hydration is to monitor the colour of your urine. If it's dark (yellow or brown) then you are dehydrated. If it's pale (yellow or clear) then you are hydrated.

One tip that I use is to fill a big 2-litre water bottle throughout the day until I hit my number. If I finish it three times then I have had my 6 litres for the day.

The first thing I do upon waking is think about my hydration. It doesn't matter how much water I've had the day before, I am always dehydrated in the morning. I drink 2 litres at breakfast (often mixed in with electrolytes or branch chain amino acids) and finish it before I get to training.

Try to start the day with a good breakfast and ample hydration. Drinking a coffee on the run isn't going to cut it.

You can't talk about hydration without mentioning alcohol. In my opinion, if you have a performance or body transformation goal, alcohol should not play a role. And booze can be the real determining factor as to whether you get OK results or great results.

I'm not suggesting you never drink again, but I advise you to think about what, how much and when you drink.

I drink in my off-season, but as soon as I want to get back into shape I cut booze completely from my diet.

Alcohol will really inhibit the fat loss process and if you over-indulge you will just end up counting a lot of wasted calories that could have come from good food.

The other thing with alcohol is it often goes hand in hand with eating badly. You get drunk, fall off the wagon and reach for the junk food. So maybe it's just best avoided.

Being well-hydrated diminishes the likelihood of muscular injury, illness, headaches and, ultimately, the chances of regression or hindered performances

MEASURING PROGRESS = BETTER RESULTS

Everything in *Cooking for Fitness* is written to help you achieve the results you want through eating.

However, to get results in the long term you simply have to track what you do in the short term.

I have talked about tracking your food daily with MyFitnessPal, but you also need to track how your body is progressing.

You need to do this for two reasons. Firstly, to keep you on track and give you confidence that what you are doing is right. Secondly, to gauge whether you need to add or take away food from your meals. If you are not gaining or losing, this can be fixed by making tweaks.

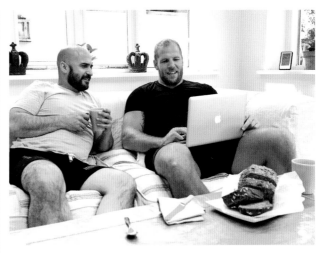

RESULTS TAKE TIME

Understand that whatever your goal, results take time. There are no quick fixes or miracles. By changing your diet and eating better you will not instantly change your body.

You will however have more energy to perform and you will recover better.

Performance on the rugby field or in your chosen sport or training is the one area that can be instantly affected by eating properly. These changes manifest themselves in all sorts of ways. I have talked about your actual performance but it could be something as simple as improved concentration.

With the body transformation side of things, it will probably take a few weeks before you start seeing changes. The way I have been taught to do it, and I believe this is the best way, is to track your progress every two weeks.

Do not track it every day. If you do this you will get all sorts of different readings and it will ultimately mess with your head.

If you need to make changes to your diet make sure you give these changes two weeks to take effect.

The golden rule to following any programme is that you need to give it time to work. Do not allow others or your frustrations to divert you from what you are trying to do. If you reach the four-week mark and see no results then it's time to reassess what you are doing food wise and with your training.

THE BEST METHODS OF TRACKING

The ways I would track my progress are as follows...

Firstly, I would take progress photos.

Ultimately, we all want to look good in the mirror, so why not use this as your visual guide?

You need to remember that when collecting data, it's about consistency. So, you need to take a photo of yourself in your underwear at the same time of day, and using the same lighting, every time you check in.

I suggest that the best time is in the morning just after you get up, before any food or liquids are in your system.

Remember these photos are not Instagram specials; they are for you to track what you are doing. Take one from the front and one from the side. Ideally, get your mate or partner to help you.

The second way to track progress is to take measurements. I would use a tape measure (the material kind) and do the following:

♦ **Waist: take your measurements at the narrowest point of the stomach.**
♦ **Upper arm: measure the circumference around the thickest part of your upper arm, commonly at the peak of biceps to peak of triceps. Do this while tensing.**
♦ **Upper leg: measure the circumference around your thigh at its widest point, usually at the midpoint between the knee and hip.**
♦ **Chest: measure the circumference around your chest at its widest point.**

Like your photo records, take your measurements every two weeks and make sure you keep everything consistent. That means doing it at the same time of day and/or wearing the same things.

Lastly, I would track your weight. I say this with hesitation as it's a dangerous game, living and breathing by what the very inconsistent scales say.

It's much more about how you look in the mirror and, for me personally, how I perform on the rugby field. How much I weigh doesn't really play a huge role in either.

For example, some rugby teams I have played for track your weight pre-match and post-match to see how much fluid you have lost. Many have stopped this practice as lads were getting on the scales, seeing they were lighter than they thought, and feeling less powerful for the game.

Remember that you can *look* far better than you do now and actually weigh *more*. Like all the other measurements I have suggested, weigh yourself once every two weeks, at the same time of day, just after you have woken up.

TIME TO ENJOY

Now you have all the info and tips, go and enjoy cooking, eating, playing and training well.

This book is about giving you some quick, simple and healthy recipes that will help you achieve your goals.

I have covered everything with a broad brushstroke within *Cooking for Fitness* to give you a taste of how simple it is to make changes to your body and lifestyle. If you want to know more, then check out my other guides and books.

Thank you so much for buying this book and for your continued support.

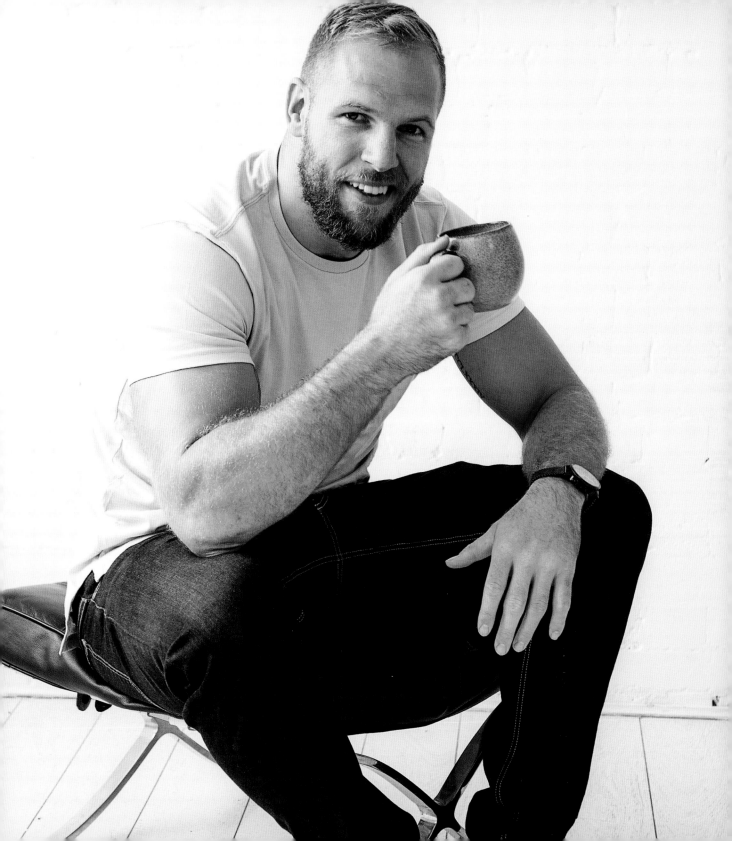

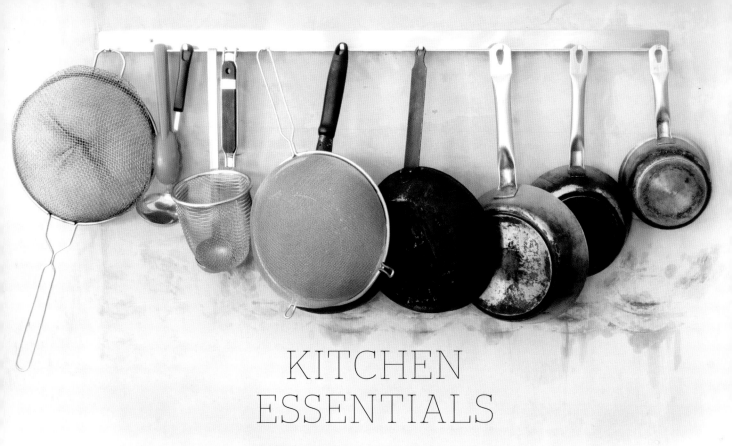

KITCHEN ESSENTIALS

EQUIPMENT TIPS: FOR BETTER COOKING

The secret to a good, structured eating pattern is efficiency in the kitchen. Don't worry, we are not expecting you to become a master chef, but with a few equipment and cupboard basics you can take control of your kitchen and your diet. Our top tips: prepare all your ingredients ahead and have them in front of you, ready to go, and clean up as you cook. It's all simple stuff, but here are a few words of guidance for anyone starting from scratch.

PANS & TRAYS

We use a range of **pans** and **trays** in this book. You'll need small (16cm), medium (18cm) and large **saucepans** (20cm), a **wok** (you can use the large saucepan at a push), small (20cm) and large (24cm) **frying pans,** a **griddle pan** (a large **frying pan** will do, but you won't drain the fats as efficiently or get the neat lines) and small, medium and large **roasting trays**. We also use a six-hole **muffin tin,** a **baking tray,** a 450g **loaf tin,** a 22-25cm **round pie dish** and a 20cm square **oven tin**.

FOOD PROCESSING & BLENDING

If you are going to make a lot of smoothies or juices, a good-quality **juicer** would be an investment and save you time, as well as get the most out of your fruit and veggies. But a **food processor** or **hand blender** will work just as well. We blend a good deal in this book – from making curry pastes to salad dressings, so if you have none of the above, you can get a decent hand blender, which will do everything, for around a tenner.

KITCHEN NOTES

FOR THE BEST RESULTS:
- Use large eggs.
- Use metric measuring spoons and scales.
- Spoonfuls are level, unless otherwise stated.
- Oven temperatures given are for non fan-assisted ovens. For fan-assisted ovens, reduce the temperatures by 10-20°C.
- Use separate chopping boards

and knives for raw meat/fish and food that is ready to eat.

NUTRITION
Nutrition is calculated as accurately as possible but may vary depending on ingredients.

SPECIAL DIETS KEY
GF = Gluten free
DF = Dairy free
V = Vegetarian
VG = Vegan

CONVERSION CHART

WEIGHT

METRIC	IMPERIAL
15g	½oz
30g	1oz
60g	2oz
85g	3oz
100g	4oz
150g	5oz
200g	7oz
225g	8oz
450g	1lb
500g	1lb 2oz
1kg	2lb 4oz

VOLUME

METRIC	IMPERIAL	USA CUPS
5ml	1 teaspoon	
15ml	1 tablespoon	
30ml	2 tablespoons	⅛ cup
50ml	2fl oz	¼ cup
75ml	2½fl oz	⅓ cup
120ml	4fl oz	½ cup
150ml	¼ pint	⅔ cup
175ml	6fl oz	¾ cup
200ml	7fl oz	1 pint
250ml	8fl oz	1 cup
400ml	14fl oz	1¾ cups
1 litre	1¾ pints	4 cups

QUICK USA CONVERSIONS

1g salt	400mg sodium
100g rice	½ cup
100g oats	¾ cup

100g flour	¾ cup
60g grated Cheddar	½ cup
100g walnut halves	1 cup

KNIVES

Using the right knives is important to get the job done. A small **paring knife** will chop the small things like chilli or garlic, and will halve an avocado and cut around the sides to remove the skin. A large **chopping knife**, or **chef's knife**, will chop larger vegetables like onions and aubergines, fresh herbs and meat. You'll also need a **bread knife** for the obvious and a **carving knife** for whole pieces of meat, like the roast chicken on page 130.

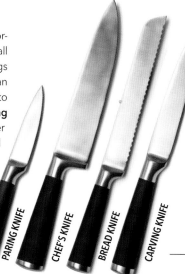

PARING KNIFE CHEF'S KNIFE BREAD KNIFE CARVING KNIFE

OTHER RECOMMENDED ITEMS

- *Kitchen scales*
- *Mixing bowls*
- *Large measuring jug*
- *Measuring spoons*
- *Chopping board*
- *Vegetable peeler*
- *Masher*
- *Ladle*
- *Slotted spoon*
- *Wooden spoons*
- *Spatula*
- *Whisk*
- *Sieve*
- *Grater*
- *Airtight lunch boxes*
- *Oven gloves*
- *Apron*

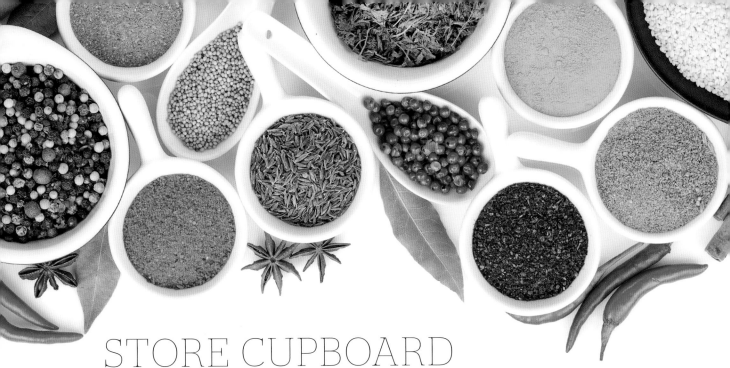

STORE CUPBOARD INGREDIENTS

HAVING THESE TO HAND WILL MAKE YOUR COOKING EASIER, TASTIER AND HEALTHIER

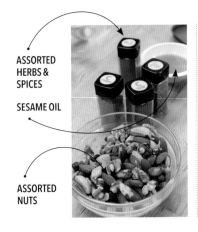

ASSORTED HERBS & SPICES

SESAME OIL

ASSORTED NUTS

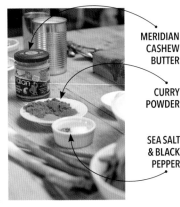

MERIDIAN CASHEW BUTTER

CURRY POWDER

SEA SALT & BLACK PEPPER

ESSENTIALS

Omar says: 'You'll need salt and freshly ground black pepper on standby for many of the recipes. Oats and brown rice are a good source of complex, slow-release carbs and, if you're a fan of risotto, then Arborio rice will ensure a perfect, creamy end result, as in our Spinach, lemon & broad bean risotto, page 166. Cocoa or cacao powder is used to flavour many of the snacks and smoothies, but make sure you go for the unsweet-ened variety.'

Salt/sea salt
Freshly ground black pepper
Garlic
Ginger
Red chillies
Oats
Brown rice
Arborio rice
Quinoa
Plain flour
Cocoa or cacao powder (unsweet-ened)
Stock pots or cubes

IN THE FRIDGE

James says: 'These are the essentials I always have in my fridge. It means I invariably have the basis of a quick, healthy meal.'

Chicken breasts
Lean minced beef (5% fat)
Eggs
Natural yoghurt
Milk
Frozen veg
Spinach
Tomatoes

TINS

Omar says: 'Tinned beans and pulses are ready to use and are a quick, low-fat way to add protein, fibre and iron to a meal, as in our Sweet potato, butter bean & avocado hash, page 64.

Butter beans
Kidney beans
Chickpeas
Chopped tomatoes
Tuna in spring water
Coconut milk

NUT BUTTERS

James says:
'Nut butters are a brilliant source of natural energy and an easy way to add flavour to a dish. I have been a fan of Meridian for many years, and an official ambassador for the last 2 years. So it's no surprise that they feature in a number of recipes within *Cooking For Fitness*.

When writing this book, and putting the recipes together with Omar, I only wanted to include foods that I personally ate and liked. The reason I like Meridian products goes beyond their brilliant flavours. Their nut butters

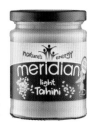

include only the most natural ingredients, are completely gluten free and contain absolutely no palm oil. These are all factors to consider when looking to really nail your diet and maximise your health.

For my own personal nutrition plan, I find that I use nut butters every day in one way or another to top up my macros, be it fats and/or proteins. On normal training days, I focus on having a good source of protein, which is usually eggs, either boiled or scrambled. My partner Chloe is an unreal cook, so

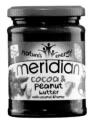

often I get some amazing creations, like Mexican eggs. I then always have porridge with Meridian nut butter in it, as well as a protein shake with oats mixed with more nut butter, for the drive to training.

The reason I add nut butters to my porridge oats every morning, is by combining these 2 food groups my body gets the complete protein hit it needs before training. The hardest macro to hit is protein, so that extra boost makes my life much easier. Consuming protein before you train is vital in preventing muscle breakdown and maximising protein synthesis. Post training, I often smear Meridian nut butters on wholegrain bread, creating a rich source of

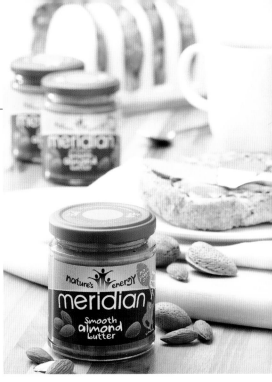

natural proteins which stimulates muscle growth and helps my body recover.

They're also great for cooking or baking, as in our Satay chicken with papaya & chilli salad, page 133, and the Banana bread with pumpkin and sunflower seeds, page 190.

And if you love chocolate, their range of nut butters with cocoa gives you a chocolatey sweet treat without

any refined sugar added.

Spread it on rice cakes or on our homebaked flapjacks, page 178.'

**Crunchy /Smooth Peanut Butters
Almond Butter
Cashew Butter
Cocoa & Hazelnut Butter
Pumpkin Seed Butter
Sunflower Seed Butter
Tahini
Yeast Extract
Molasses
Pure Cane
Date Syrup**

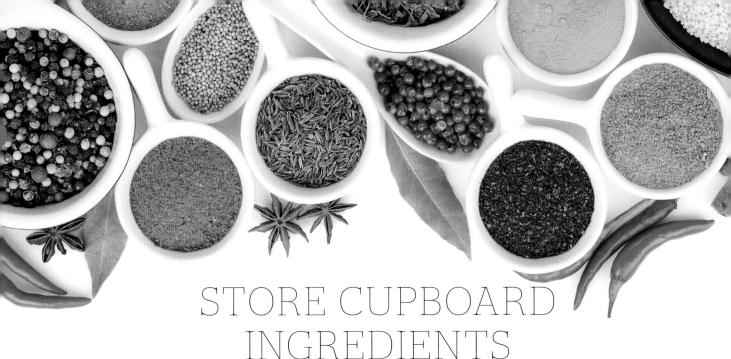

STORE CUPBOARD INGREDIENTS

SAUCES

Omar says:
'Having a good range of sauces in the cupboard will add a depth of flavour to your dishes. For example, adding a dash of Tabasco and Worcestershire sauce to the tomato salad on page 91 will make the flavours zing out.'

Dijon mustard
Tabasco sauce
Worcestershire sauce
Soy sauce
Tomato passata

OILS & VINEGARS

Omar says: 'For most of our savoury dishes, olive oil is the healthiest option, however rapeseed oil is a good alternative. Coconut oil has a mild coconut flavour that suits curries and sweet snacks, as in our Banana & almond seedy bars, page 176.'

Olive oil
Sesame oil
Coconut oil
Balsamic vinegar
White wine vinegar

DRIED HERBS & SPICES

Omar says: 'It's well worth investing in herbs and spices as they are the key to exciting and delicious dishes. It does make some of the ingredients lists in the recipes look longer, but throwing in a few herbs and spices is an amazingly easy way of adding flavour to your meals.'

Sage
Oregano
Ground cumin
Dried chilli flakes
Cajun seasoning
Paprika
Smoked paprika
Curry powder
Ground cinnamon
Turmeric
Ground nutmeg
Ground coriander

NUTS & SEEDS

James says: 'While they may be high in calories, nuts contain essential fatty acids that the human body needs to achieve and maintain optimum health. While essential fatty acids should only be included in small amounts (to avoid slipping into a calorie surplus), they should absolutely be part of your daily diet. Nuts combined with grains create a complete protein.'

Almonds
Ground almonds
Brazil nuts
Cashews
Hazelnuts
Pistachios
Walnuts
Mixed nuts
Linseeds
Sunflower seeds
Pumpkin seeds

FRESH FRUIT & VEGETABLES

James says: 'It's important to keep a good selection of healthy fruit and veg. Here are some of my favourites.'

Apples
Bananas
Blueberries
Strawberries
Limes
Lemons
Tomatoes
Avocados
Red onions
Beetroot
Carrots
Broccoli
Sweet potatoes

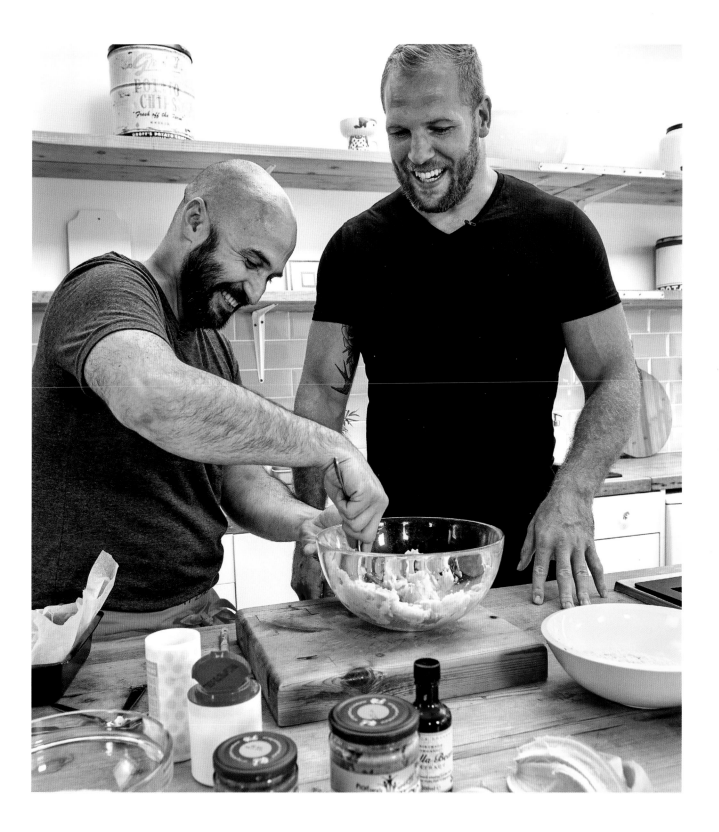

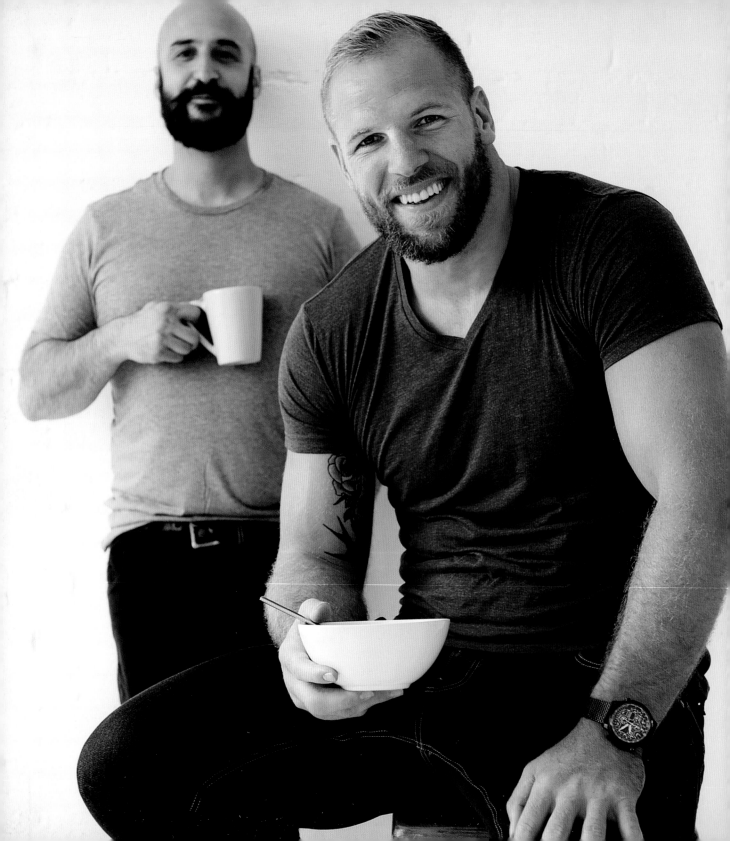

1

LOW-CARB BREAKFASTS

Whether they're based on
eggs, fish or yoghurt, these
high-protein, low-carb
breakfasts are how I start the day
when I'm looking to reduce my
body fat and get leaner.

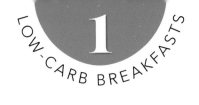
BAKED EGGS WITH KALE, SPINACH & PARMESAN

SERVES **2** ◆ PREP TIME **5 MINS** ◆ COOK TIME **30 MINS** ◆ DIFFICULTY **EASY** ◆ **GF**

INGREDIENTS

1 knob of butter
1 large handful curly kale, tough stalks removed
2 large handfuls baby spinach leaves
200ml tomato passata
4 large eggs
½ avocado, chopped
2 tablespoons finely grated Parmesan cheese

JAMES SAYS: 'Eggs are my go-to breakfast, especially on training days.'

METHOD

1. Preheat your oven to 200°C.

2. Melt the butter in a medium-sized saucepan over a medium heat. Toss in the kale and season with salt and pepper. Cook the kale until it begins to wilt. Now add the spinach and remove from the heat, but continue to stir until the spinach wilts. Tip into a colander and allow to drain.

3. Place the kale and spinach in the bottom of a small roasting tray, spoon over the passata sauce. Crack the eggs over the passata sauce and season each one with salt and pepper.

4. Scatter the avocado over the top of the eggs, then sprinkle over the Parmesan cheese.

5. Bake in the oven for 12 minutes or until the whites of the eggs are cooked through. Serve.

PER SERVING

CARBS	ENERGY	FAT	SATURATES	PROTEIN	SUGAR	FIBRE	SALT
5.5g	403 kcal	29g	10.5g	27.5g	5g	3g	1g

6 69014 44873 6

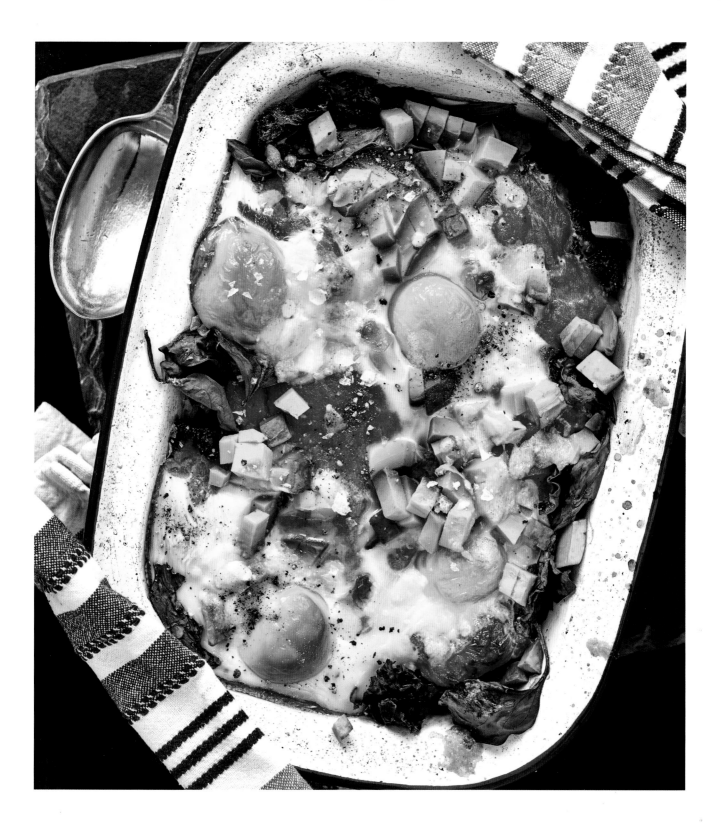

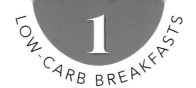

BEETROOT & MACKEREL FRITTATA

SERVES **2** ◆ PREP TIME **10 MINS** ◆ COOK TIME **15 MINS** ◆ DIFFICULTY **EASY** ◆ **GF** ◆ **DF**

INGREDIENTS

6 large eggs
1 fillet smoked mackerel, finely sliced
4 small cooked beetroots, sliced
1 small bunch watercress, roughly chopped

JAMES SAYS: 'The mackerel in this dish makes it rich in healthy omega 3 fats.'

METHOD

1. Preheat your oven to 180°C. Crack the eggs into a large jug and season with salt and pepper. Whisk the eggs well.

2. Place the mackerel, beetroot and watercress in an oven-proof frying pan, ensuring that all the ingredients are spread evenly throughout the pan. Pour the eggs over the top.

3. Place the pan into the oven and bake for 15 minutes, or until the frittata is cooked through. Allow to rest for 5 minutes before slicing and serving.

PER SERVING

CARBS	ENERGY	FAT	SATURATES	PROTEIN	SUGAR	FIBRE	SALT
5g	460 kcal	31g	8g	39g	5g	2g	1.9g

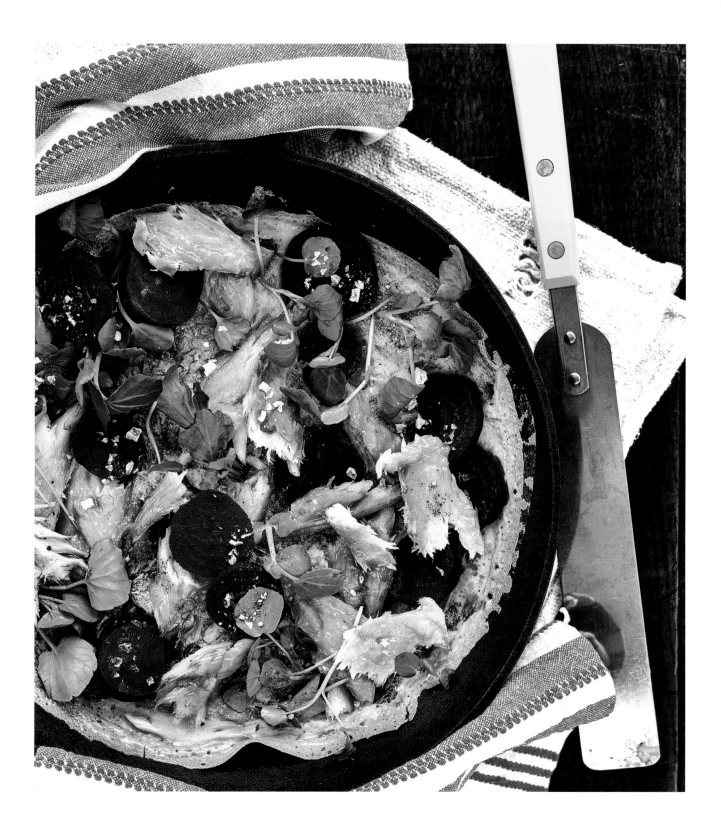

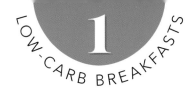

SMOKED TROUT WITH AVOCADO & COTTAGE CHEESE WITH SEEDS

SERVES **2** ◆ PREP TIME **10 MINS** ◆ DIFFICULTY **VERY EASY** ◆ **GF**

INGREDIENTS
100g smoked trout
Juice of ½ lemon
4 tablespoons cottage cheese
1 avocado, peeled and sliced
2 tablespoons omega seeds

OMAR SAYS: 'Add eggs of your choice for extra protein.'

METHOD
1. Divide the trout between two serving plates. Mill a little black pepper over the trout then squeeze over the juice of the lemon.
2. Divide the cottage cheese and avocado slices between the two plates. Sprinkle over the omega seeds and serve.

PER SERVING

CARBS	ENERGY	FAT	SATURATES	PROTEIN	SUGAR	FIBRE	SALT
3.5g	333 kcal	26g	6g	18.5g	1.5g	5g	1.3g

6 69014 44875 0

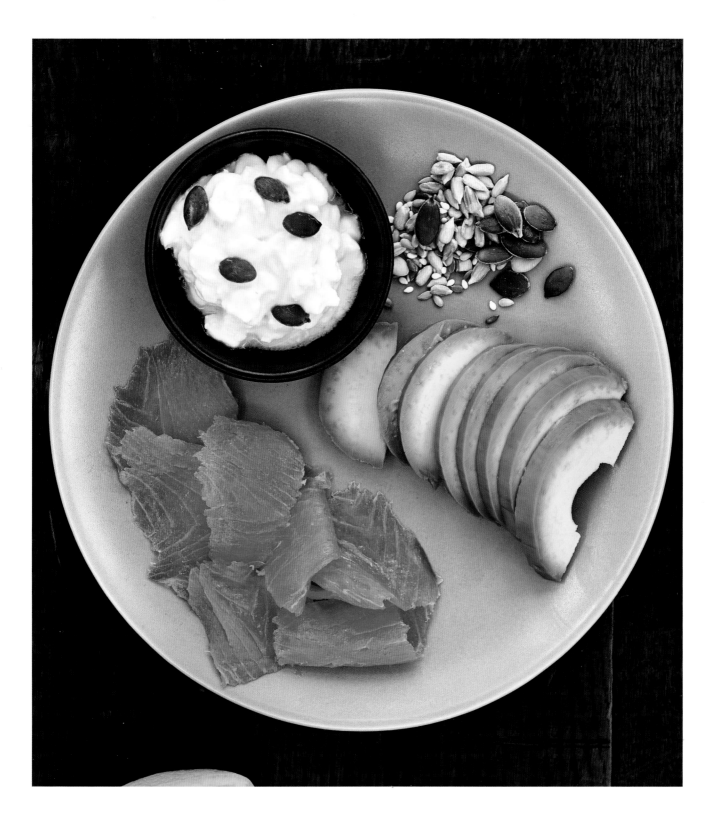

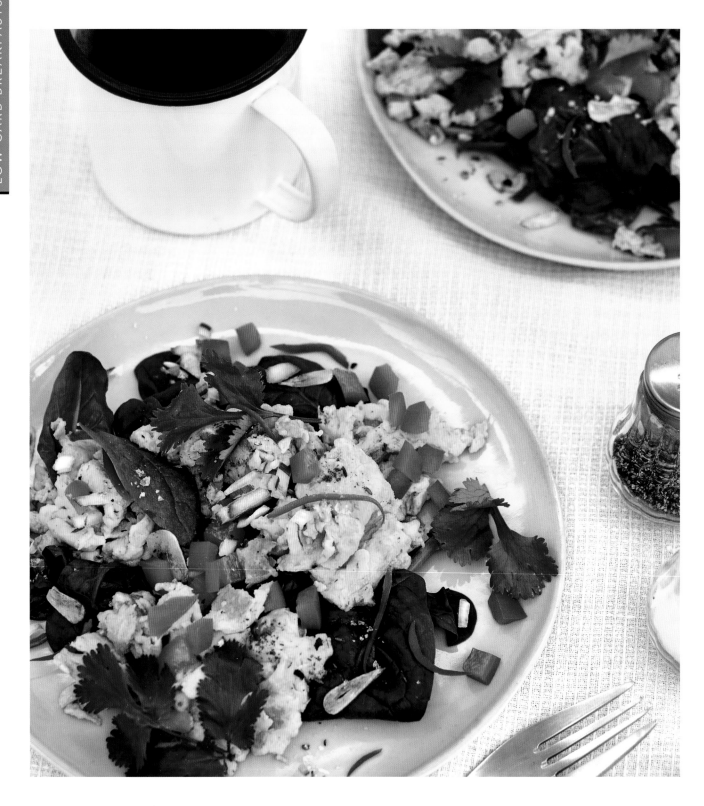

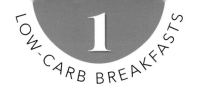
SPICY OAXACA SCRAMBLED EGGS WITH SPINACH

SERVES **2** ◆ PREP TIME **10 MINS** ◆ COOK TIME **10 MINS** ◆ DIFFICULTY **EASY** ◆ **GF** ◆ **DF** ◆ **V**

INGREDIENTS

¼ red onion, finely chopped
1 small bunch coriander, chopped
½ red pepper, finely chopped
6 large eggs
1 pinch ground cumin
1 garlic clove, finely sliced
½ red chilli, finely sliced
1 handful baby spinach leaves

OMAR SAYS: 'This recipe is from Oaxaca in Mexico and has a tasty chilli kick.'

METHOD

1. Mix together the red onion, coriander and red pepper in a medium bowl and set aside.

2. Crack the eggs into a medium bowl and season with salt and pepper and cumin. Whisk the eggs well. Stir in the garlic and chilli.

3. Pour the eggs into a medium saucepan and place over a medium heat. Cook the eggs for 5-6 minutes, stirring all the time. Once the eggs are cooked, remove from the heat and fold in the spinach leaves. Keep stirring the eggs and the spinach will wilt. Now stir in the red pepper mix. Divide between two serving plates and serve.

PER SERVING

CARBS	ENERGY	FAT	SATURATES	PROTEIN	SUGAR	FIBRE	SALT
3.5g	308 kcal	19g	5g	28g	3g	3.5g	0.9g

6 69014 44876 7

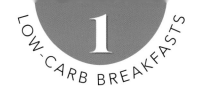

GRAB & GO YOGHURT POTS

MANGO, PASSION FRUIT & LIME

SERVES **2** ◆ PREP TIME **10 MINS** ◆ DIFFICULTY **VERY EASY** ◆ **GF** ◆ **V**

INGREDIENTS

½ mango
1 passion fruit
Zest and juice of 1 lime
300ml Greek yoghurt
1 teaspoon honey

METHOD

1. Finely dice the mango flesh and place in a mixing bowl. Slice the passion fruit in half, scoop out the seeds and mix with the mango. Add the zest and lime juice to the mango.
2. Divide the yoghurt between two serving bowls and spoon over the mango mix. Drizzle over the honey and serve.

PER SERVING

CARBS	ENERGY	FAT	SATURATES	PROTEIN	SUGAR	FIBRE	SALT
17.5g	**262 kcal**	**16.5g**	**10.5g**	**10g**	**16.5g**	**2g**	**0.25g**

6 69014 44877 4

DARK CHOCOLATE, PECAN, ALMOND & HONEY

SERVES **2** ◆ PREP TIME **5 MINS** ◆ DIFFICULTY **VERY EASY** ◆ **GF** ◆ **V**

INGREDIENTS

300ml Greek yoghurt
1 tablespoon dark chocolate pieces
1 tablespoon pecan nuts
1 tablespoon flaked almonds
1 teaspoon honey

METHOD

1. Divide the yoghurt between two serving bowls. Sprinkle over the chocolate pieces, pecan nuts and almonds. Drizzle over the honey and serve.

PER SERVING

CARBS	ENERGY	FAT	SATURATES	PROTEIN	SUGAR	FIBRE	SALT
15g	**350 kcal**	**27g**	**12g**	**11.5g**	**14.5g**	**1g**	**0.25g**

6 69014 44878 1

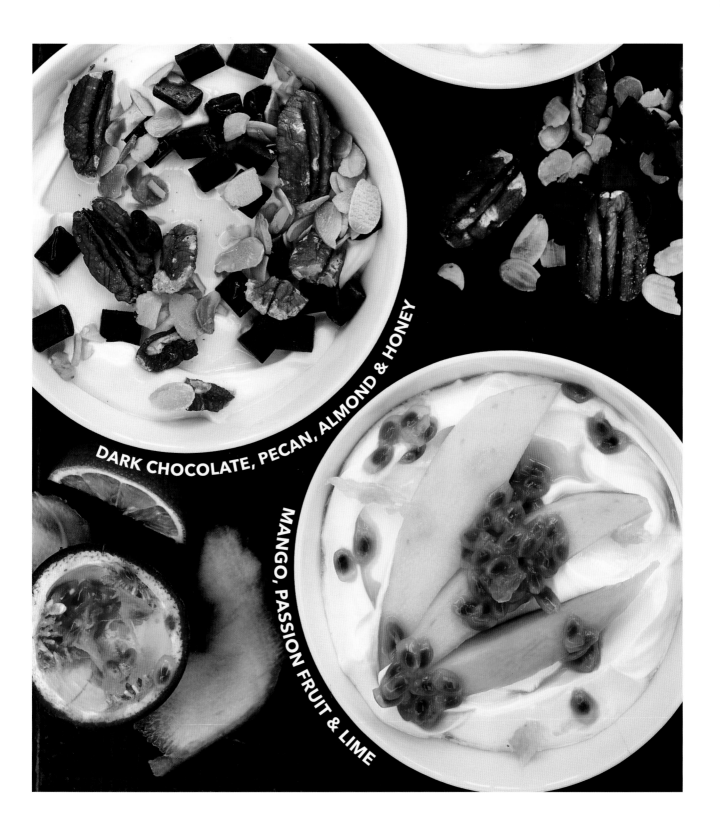

DARK CHOCOLATE, PECAN, ALMOND & HONEY

MANGO, PASSION FRUIT & LIME

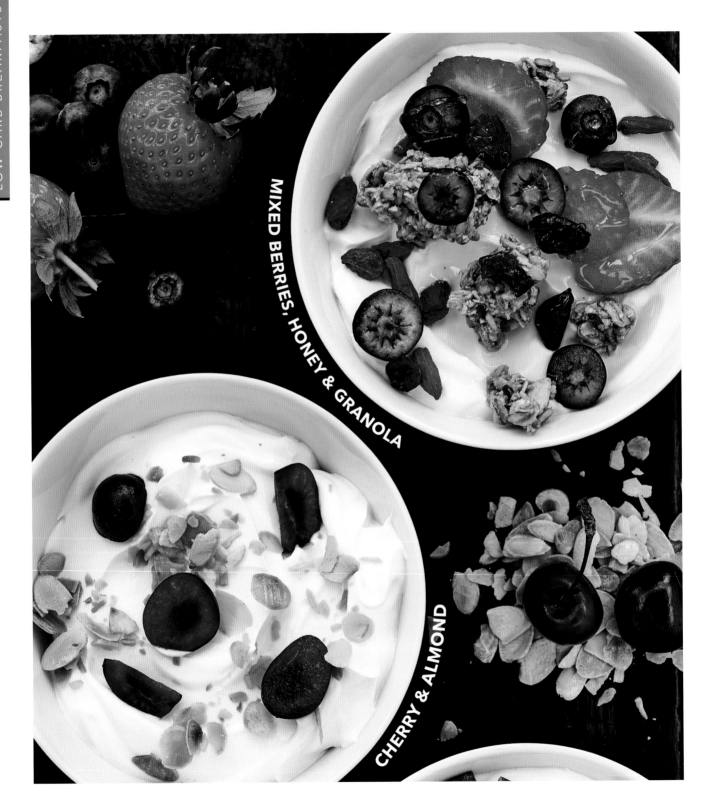

MIXED BERRIES, HONEY & GRANOLA

CHERRY & ALMOND

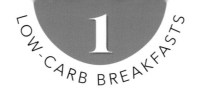
GRAB & GO
YOGHURT POTS

MIXED BERRIES, HONEY & GRANOLA

SERVES **2** ◆ PREP TIME **5 MINS** ◆ DIFFICULTY **VERY EASY** ◆ **V**

INGREDIENTS
300ml Greek yoghurt
3 strawberries
1 tablespoon blueberries
1 teaspoon dried cranberries
1 teaspoon goji berries
1 tablespoon granola
1 teaspoon honey

METHOD
1. Divide the yoghurt between two serving bowls. Remove the stalks from the strawberries, cut them into quarters and place them on top of the yoghurt. Scatter the blueberries, cranberries, goji berries and granola over the top. Drizzle over the honey and serve.

PER SERVING

CARBS	ENERGY	FAT	SATURATES	PROTEIN	SUGAR	FIBRE	SALT
19g	266 kcal	17g	10.5g	9.5g	15.5g	1.5g	0.4g

6 69014 44879 8

CHERRY & ALMOND

SERVES **2** ◆ PREP TIME **5 MINS** ◆ DIFFICULTY **VERY EASY** ◆ **GF** ◆ **V**

INGREDIENTS
100g fresh cherries
300ml Greek yoghurt
1 tablespoon flaked almonds
1 teaspoon honey

METHOD
1. Remove the cherry stones and discard. Slice the cherries in half.
2. Divide the yoghurt between two serving bowls and top with the cherries. Sprinkle over the almonds, drizzle over the honey and serve.

PER SERVING

CARBS	ENERGY	FAT	SATURATES	PROTEIN	SUGAR	FIBRE	SALT
16g	283 kcal	19.5g	10.5g	11g	15g	0.5g	0.25g

6 69014 44880 4

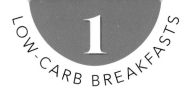

AVOCADO, HAM & CHILLI TARTS

SERVES **2** ◆ PREP TIME **10 MINS** ◆ COOK TIME **20 MINS** ◆ DIFFICULTY **EASY** ◆ **GF** ◆ **DF**

INGREDIENTS

4 large eggs
1 avocado, peeled and chopped
½ red chilli, finely chopped
½ small bunch coriander, finely chopped
6 slices Parma ham

JAMES SAYS: 'If I'm eating on the go, I bake these tarts in muffin cases rather than straight in the tin and take them to training.'

METHOD

1. Preheat your oven to 200°C.
2. Crack the eggs into a medium bowl and season with salt and pepper. Whisk well.
3. Place the avocado in a medium-sized bowl. Stir in the chilli and coriander.
4. Line a muffin tin with the Parma ham. Divide the avocado mix between the ham cases. Pour over the eggs and bake in the oven for 20 minutes or until cooked through. Allow to rest for 5 minutes before serving.

PER SERVING

CARBS	ENERGY	FAT	SATURATES	PROTEIN	SUGAR	FIBRE	SALT
1.5g	400 kcal	31g	8g	27g	0.5g	3.5g	2g

6 69014 44881 1

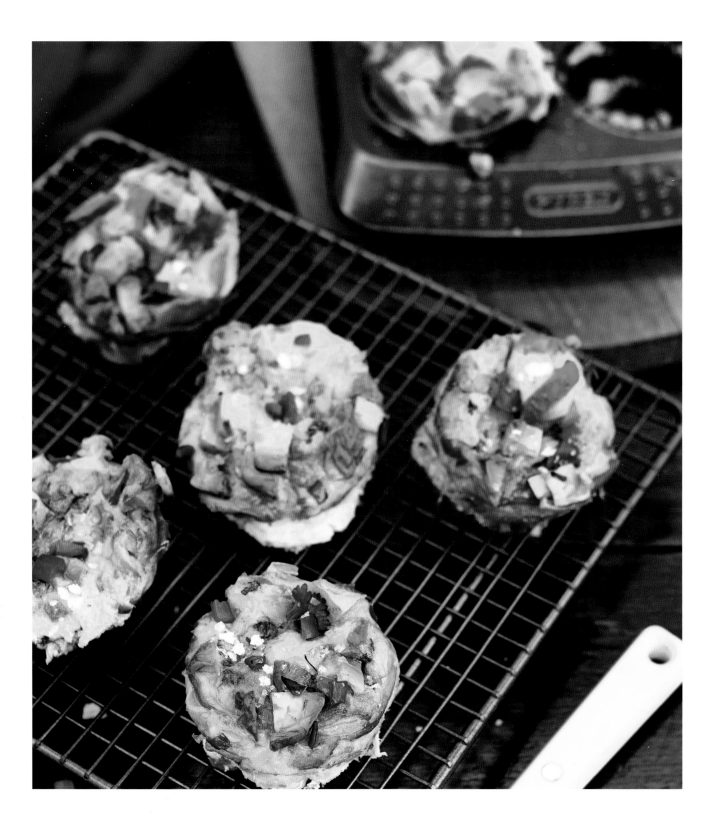

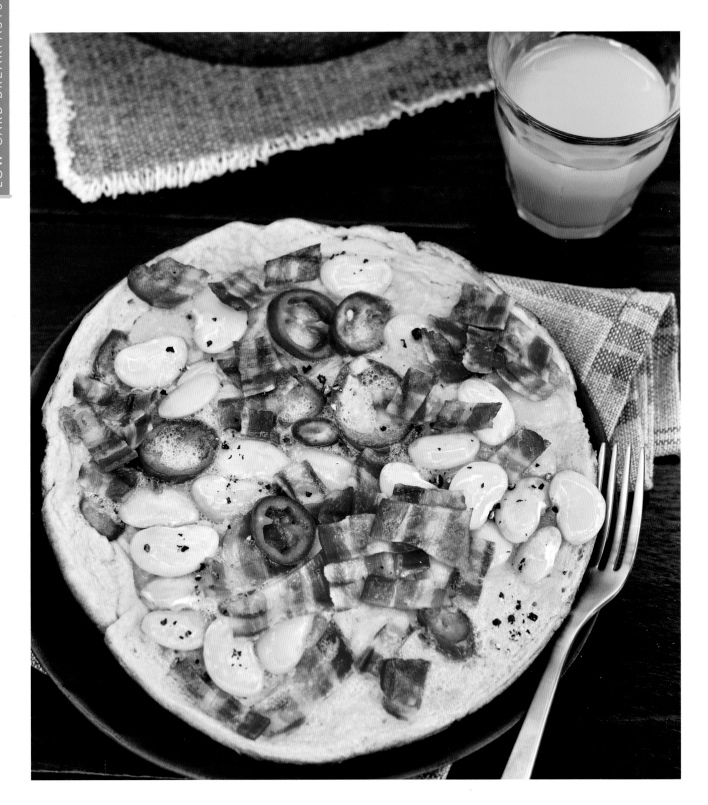

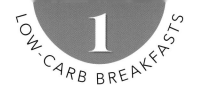
BACON, JALAPENO & BUTTER BEAN OMELETTE

SERVES **1** ◆ PREP TIME **10 MINS** ◆ COOK TIME **15 MINS** ◆ DIFFICULTY **EASY** ◆ **GF**

INGREDIENTS

2 slices streaky bacon
4 slices pickled jalapeno chilli or
½ fresh green chilli, finely chopped
3 large eggs
1 knob of butter
50g cooked butter beans

OMAR SAYS: 'For a lower-fat option, use lean bacon instead of streaky.'

METHOD

1. Preheat the grill to high. Place the bacon on a tray and cook under the grill for 7-8 minutes or until cooked through. Allow to cool before slicing into strips ½cm thick and set aside. Stir in the jalapeno chilli.

2. Crack the eggs into a bowl and season with salt and pepper. Whisk the eggs well. Heat a frying pan over a medium heat and add the butter. Pour the eggs into the pan and cook the omelette for 2 minutes or until it has started to set on the bottom. Now sprinkle the bacon and jalapeno over the omelette and top with the butter beans. Pop under the grill for 30 seconds. Turn out onto a plate and serve immediately.

PER SERVING

CARBS	ENERGY	FAT	SATURATES	PROTEIN	SUGAR	FIBRE	SALT
9.5g	514kcal	35g	12g	38g	1.5g	4g	2.8g

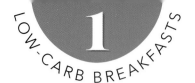

HOMEMADE SAUSAGES, EGGS & AVOCADO

SERVES **2** ◆ PREP TIME **15 MINS** ◆ COOK TIME **25 MINS** ◆ DIFFICULTY **EASY** ◆ **GF** ◆ **DF**

INGREDIENTS

300g lean minced pork
4 sage leaves, finely chopped
or 2 teaspoons dried sage
½ teaspoon ground cumin
1 avocado, peeled and chopped
Juice of 1 lime
1 teaspoon dried chilli flakes
1 teaspoon white wine vinegar
2 eggs

JAMES SAYS: 'The beauty of homemade sausages is that you know exactly what's in them.'

METHOD

1. Preheat your oven to 200°C.

2. Place the minced pork in a medium mixing bowl and mix in the sage. Add the cumin and season with salt and pepper. Give the pork a gentle mix and shape into 6 sausages. Place them on a plate and pop into the fridge for 30 minutes.

3. Place the avocado in a small mixing bowl, squeeze over the lime juice and add the chilli flakes. With a fork gently mash the avocado. Set aside.

4. Half-fill a small pan of water and bring to the boil then turn down to a simmer.

5. Place the pork sausages on a tray and bake in the oven for 15 minutes or until cooked through. Allow to rest for 2-3 minutes.

6. Add the vinegar to the water and gently crack the eggs into it. Cook the eggs for 3-4 minutes before draining. To serve, spoon the avocado onto a plate and top with the eggs, with the sausages alongside.

PER SERVING

CARBS	ENERGY	FAT	SATURATES	PROTEIN	SUGAR	FIBRE	SALT
3g	464 kcal	29g	8g	47g	0.5g	3.5g	0.6g

6 69014 44883 5

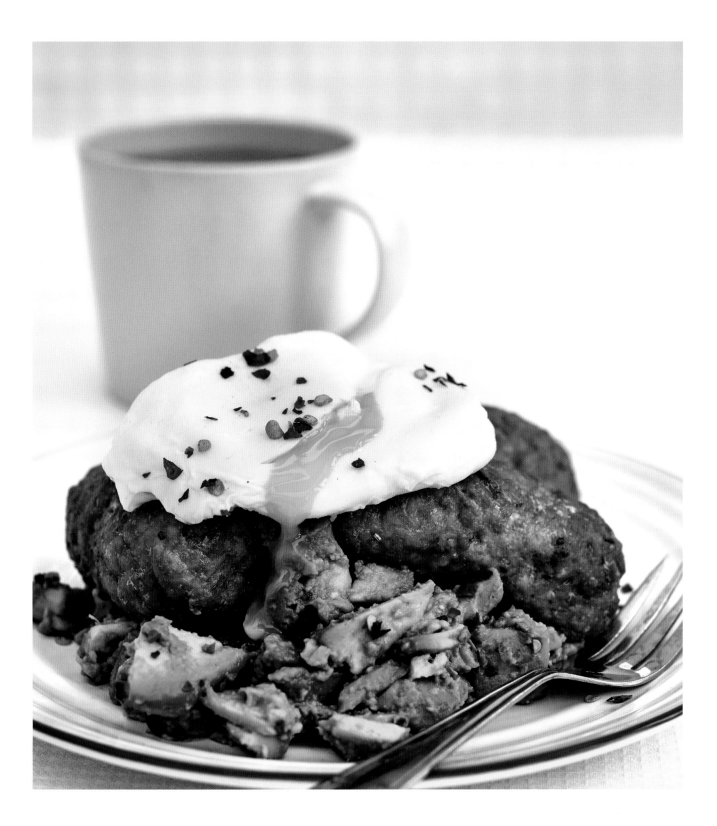

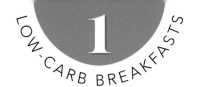
SUPER GREENS SMOOTHIE

SERVES **3-4** ◆ PREP TIME **10 MINS** ◆ COOK TIME **30 MINS** ◆ DIFFICULTY **VERY EASY** ◆ **GF** ◆ **DF** ◆ **VG**

INGREDIENTS

1 green apple
½ cucumber
1 celery stalk
4 kale leaves, stalks removed
2 handfuls baby spinach leaves
240ml water
120ml almond milk
120ml coconut water
Juice of 1 lime

OMAR SAYS: 'This smoothie would be great with a little green chilli too.'

METHOD

1. Remove the core from the apple. Roughly chop the apple, cucumber and celery. Place them in a food processor along with the remaining ingredients and blend until smooth and serve.

PER SERVING

CARBS	ENERGY	FAT	SATURATES	PROTEIN	SUGAR	FIBRE	SALT
6.5g	48 kcal	1.5g	0.2g	2g	6.5g	1.5g	0.2g

6 69014 44884 2

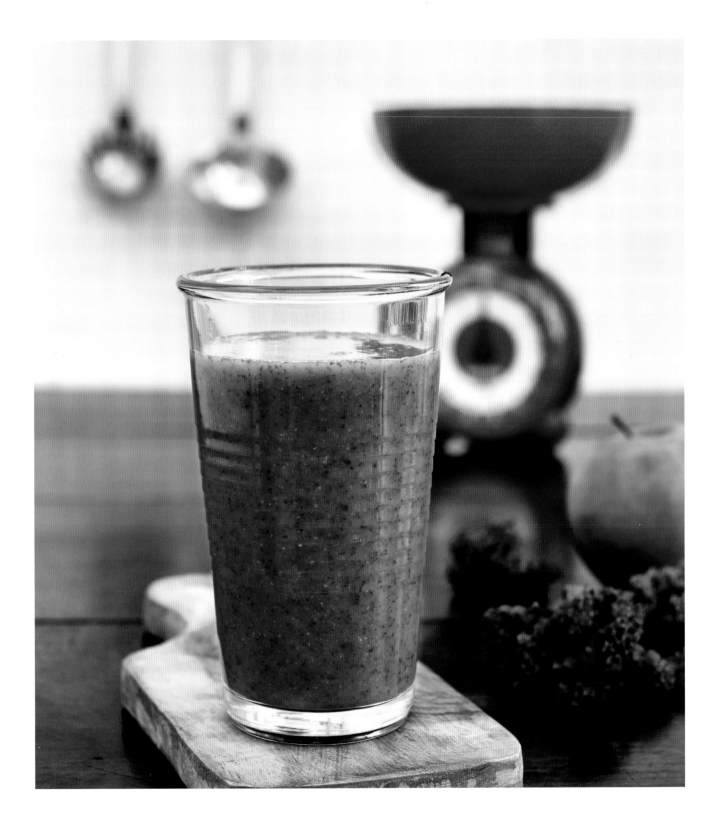

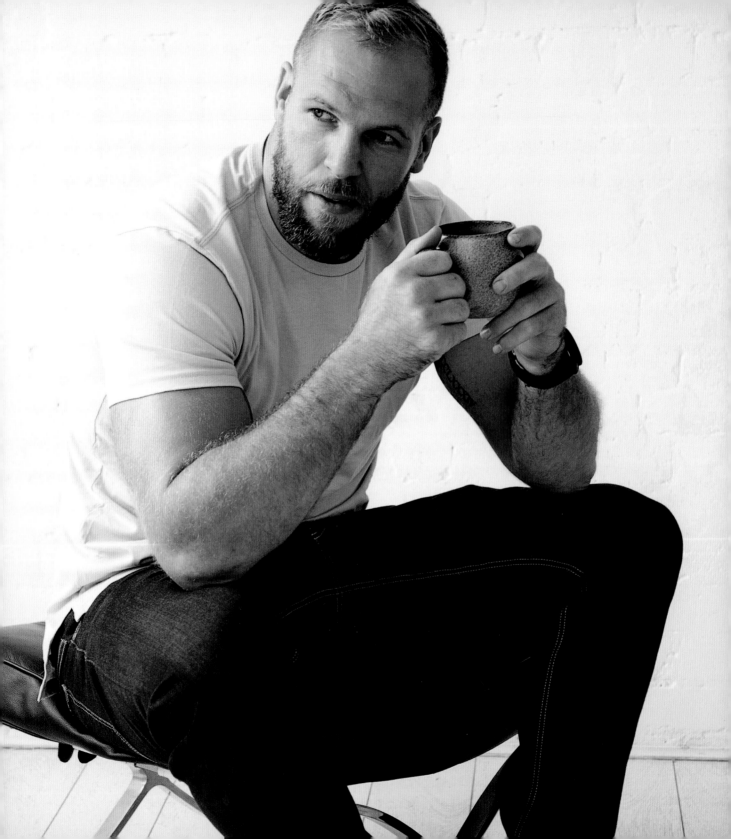

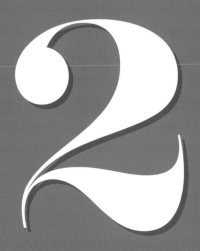

2

HIGH-CARB
BREAKFASTS

"

If you are physically active,
and especially if you are a
performance athlete, carbs need
to play a starring role in your diet.
But your level of activity has to
match your intake.

"

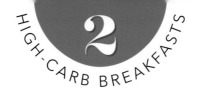

BANANA & PEANUT BUTTER FRENCH TOAST

SERVES **2** ◆ PREP TIME **5 MINS** ◆ COOK TIME **10 MINS** ◆ DIFFICULTY **EASY** ◆ **V**

INGREDIENTS

2 bananas
2 tablespoons caster sugar
2 large eggs
2 knobs of butter
4 slices brioche
2 tablespoons cherry jam
2 tablespoons Meridian Peanut Butter
2 tablespoons Greek yoghurt
100g fresh pitted cherries, halved

JAMES SAYS: 'This indulgent take on French toast is delicious but best eaten as an occasional treat.'

METHOD

1. Preheat your grill to high. Cut the bananas in half, then slice them lengthways into pieces roughly 1cm thick. Place on an oven tray and sprinkle over the caster sugar. Pop under the grill and cook until the sugar has caramelised. Allow to cool and set aside.

2. Crack the eggs into a bowl and whisk well. Melt the butter in a frying pan over a medium heat. Once the butter is bubbling away, dip the brioche slices into the egg one at a time and then place in the pan. Cook for 1 minute on each side or until golden brown. Remove from the pan and divide between two plates.

3. Top the French toast with the cherry jam, peanut butter and Greek yoghurt. Place the bananas on top, scatter over the fresh cherries and serve immediately.

PER SERVING

CARBS	ENERGY	FAT	SATURATES	PROTEIN	SUGAR	FIBRE	SALT
83g	649kcal	25g	10g	21g	57g	4.5g	0.9g

6 69014 44885 9

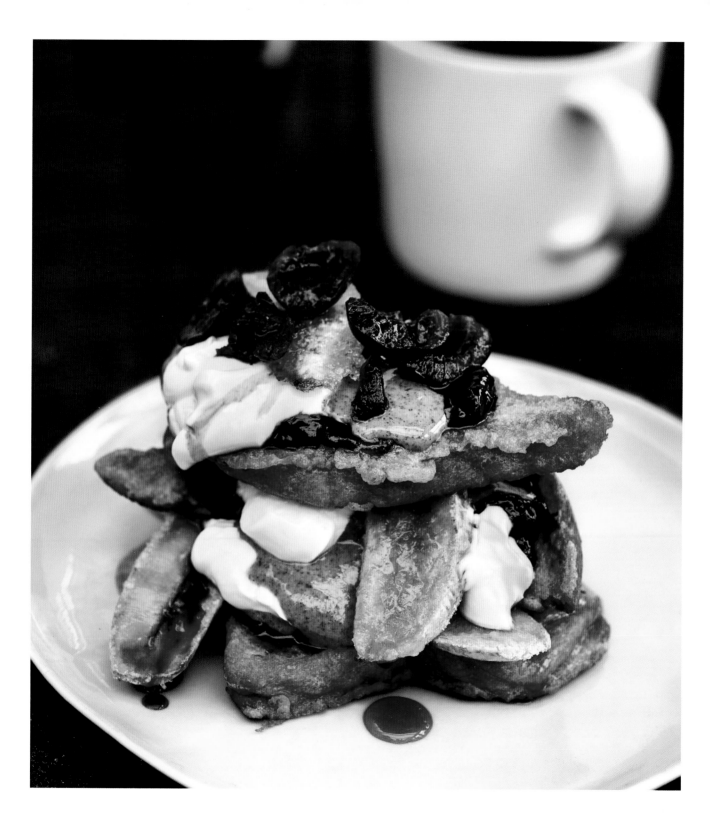

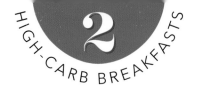

SWEET POTATO, BUTTER BEAN & AVOCADO HASH

SERVES **2** ◆ PREP TIME **10 MINS** ◆ COOK TIME **30 MINS** ◆ DIFFICULTY **EASY** ◆ **GF** ◆ **DF** ◆ **V**

INGREDIENTS

1 large sweet potato, cut into 2cm dice
1 red onion, chopped
1 tablespoon olive oil
400g tin cooked butter beans
1 small green chilli, finely chopped
1 avocado, roughly chopped
6 tablespoons tomato passata
4 large eggs

JAMES SAYS: 'The carbs and healthy fats in this breakfast will give you loads of energy on training days.'

METHOD

1. Preheat your oven to 180°C.

2. Place the sweet potato and red onion in a medium roasting tray. Season with salt and pepper and mix in the olive oil. Roast in the oven for 20 minutes or until the potato is cooked through.

3. Now add the butter beans, chilli and avocado to the tray. Pour over the passata and give it all a good mix. Crack the eggs over the top and bake in the oven for 10 minutes or until the whites of the eggs are cooked through. Serve immediately.

PER SERVING

CARBS	ENERGY	FAT	SATURATES	PROTEIN	SUGAR	FIBRE	SALT
65g	727 kcal	34g	8g	30g	19g	19g	0.8g

6 69014 44886 6

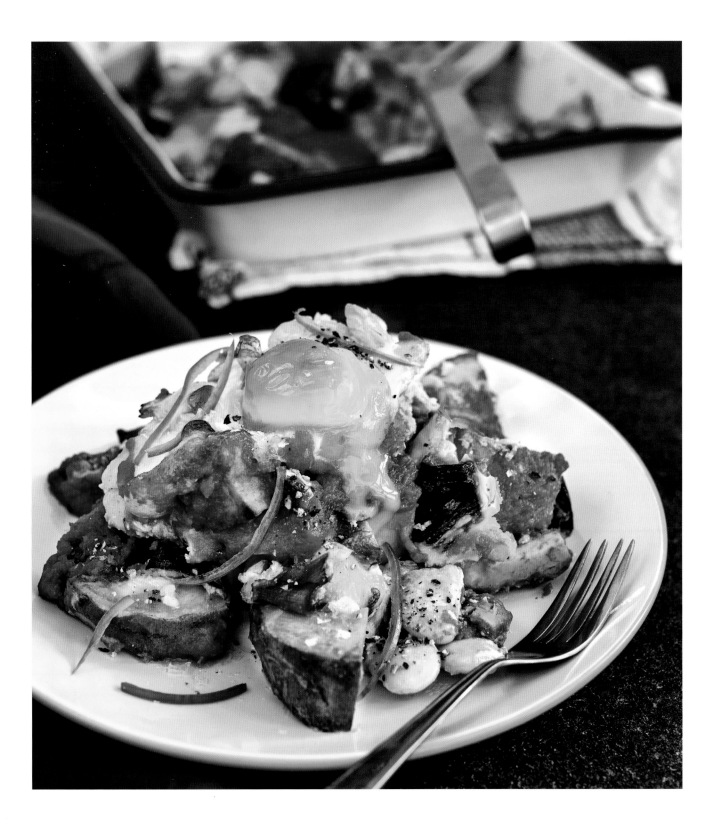

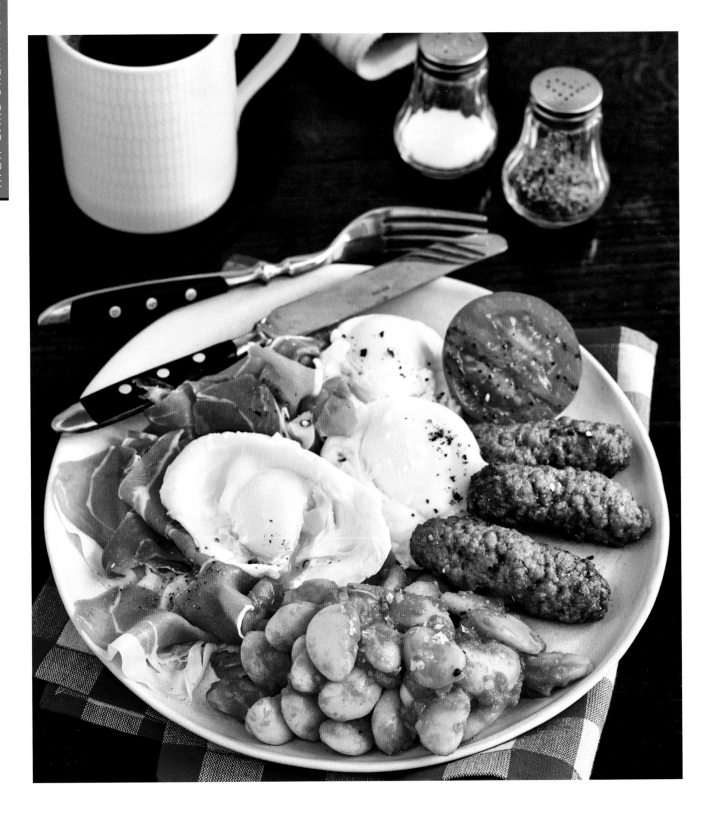

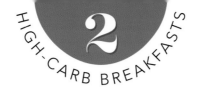
JAMES'S FULL ENGLISH BREAKFAST

SERVES **2** ◆ PREP TIME **10 MINS** ◆ COOK TIME **30 MINS** ◆ DIFFICULTY **EASY** ◆ **GF** ◆ **DF**

INGREDIENTS

300g minced pork
2 sage leaves, finely chopped
400g tin cooked butter beans
250ml tomato passata
2 plum tomatoes, halved
2 teaspoons white wine vinegar
4 large eggs
4 slices Parma ham

OMAR SAYS: 'If you need extra carbs, add one or two slices of wholemeal toast.'

METHOD

1. Preheat your oven to 180°C.

2. First make the sausages. Mix together the minced pork and the sage in a bowl. Season with salt and pepper. Shape the pork into 4 sausages and pop into the fridge for 30 minutes.

3. Cook the beans and passata sauce in a small saucepan over a low heat for 10-12 minutes. Season with salt and pepper.

4. Place the sausages on a small roasting tray and bake in the oven for 10-12 minutes or until cooked through. Meanwhile, place the tomatoes on another tray and bake in the oven for 8 minutes or until softened.

5. Half-fill a medium saucepan with water and bring to the boil. Turn down to a simmer and add the vinegar. Gently crack the eggs into the water and cook for 3 minutes.

6. Divide the eggs between 2 plates and serve with the Parma ham, tomatoes, sausages and beans.

PER SERVING

CARBS	ENERGY	FAT	SATURATES	PROTEIN	SUGAR	FIBRE	SALT
25g	644 kcal	31g	10g	62g	11g	9g	1.95g

6 69014 44887 3

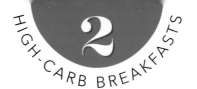

MEXICAN CHORIZO BREAKFAST BURRITO

SERVES **4** ◆ PREP TIME **5 MINS** ◆ COOK TIME **20 MINS** ◆ DIFFICULTY **EASY**

INGREDIENTS

75g cooking chorizo sausage
1 red pepper, sliced
4 eggs
1 handful baby spinach
100g tinned kidney beans
30g mature Cheddar, grated
½ teaspoon Cajun spice
1 teaspoon smoked paprika
4 tortilla wraps

OMAR SAYS: 'You could use ready-to-eat sliced chorizo instead.'

METHOD

1. Preheat your oven to 200°C.

2. Chop the chorizo sausage into pieces roughly 1cm thick and place on a roasting tray. Add the red pepper. Bake in the oven for 3 minutes or until the chorizo is cooked through.

3. Crack the eggs into a bowl and season with salt and pepper. Whisk well. Pour the eggs into a medium saucepan and cook over a medium heat. Stir continuously until the scrambled eggs are cooked. Transfer to a mixing bowl and add the spinach. Keep stirring until the spinach has wilted. Now add the kidney beans, Cheddar, Cajun spice, smoked paprika and chorizo and red pepper. Give it all a gentle stir.

4. Lay out the wraps on a work surface and spoon the mixture down the centre of the wraps. Now roll up the wraps nice and tightly. Transfer them to a roasting tin and heat in the oven for 5 minutes. Divide between two plates and serve immediately.

PER SERVING

CARBS	ENERGY	FAT	SATURATES	PROTEIN	SUGAR	FIBRE	SALT
41.5g	432kcal	18.5g	7g	22g	3g	5.5g	2.1g

6 69014 44888 0

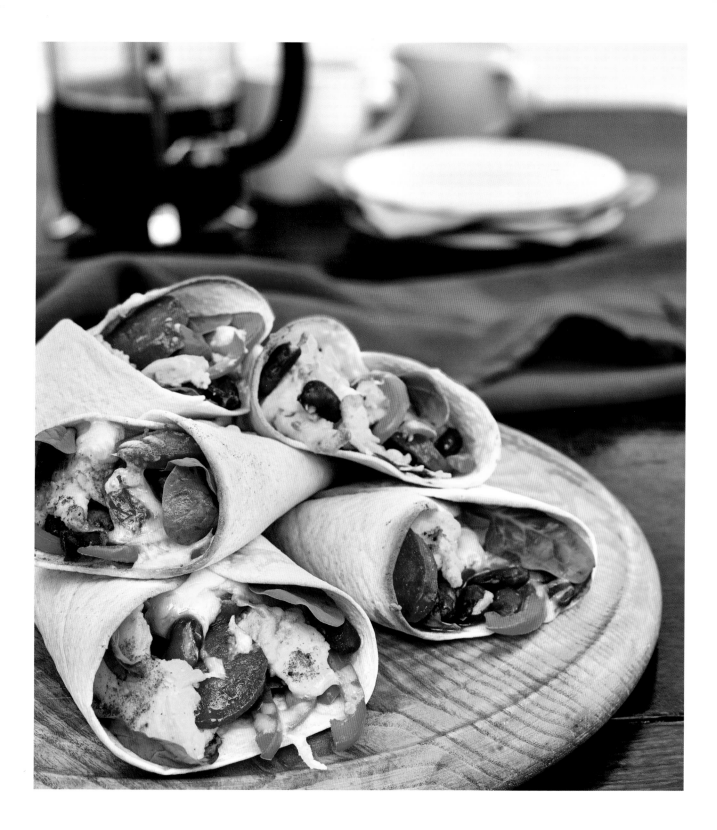

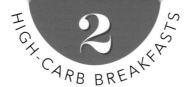

BREAKFAST BRUSCHETTA

SERVES **2** ◆ PREP TIME **10 MINS** ◆ COOK TIME **10 MINS** ◆ DIFFICULTY **EASY**

INGREDIENTS

4 slices sourdough bread
4 plum tomatoes, sliced
1 tablespoon olive oil
1 garlic clove, finely sliced
1 knob of butter
2 handfuls baby spinach
2 tablespoons cottage cheese
2 slices of ham
50g mature Cheddar, grated

JAMES SAYS: 'This makes a really quick and tasty brunch before I head out to training.'

METHOD

1. Preheat your grill to high.

2. Toast the sourdough bread under the grill on both sides.

3. Place the tomatoes on a roasting tray. Season with salt and pepper and drizzle over the olive oil. Sprinkle the garlic over the tomatoes. Pop the tray under the grill for 2-3 minutes, just until the tomatoes start to become soft.

4. Heat the butter and spinach with a pinch of pepper in a medium saucepan over a high heat. Cook the spinach for 1 minute or until wilted.

5. Spread the cottage cheese over the toast and top with the sliced tomatoes. Top the tomatoes with the spinach. Tear the ham over the spinach and sprinkle over the Cheddar cheese. Pop the bruschetta back under the grill for 1 minute or until the Cheddar has melted.

PER SERVING

CARBS	ENERGY	FAT	SATURATES	PROTEIN	SUGAR	FIBRE	SALT
46g	466kcal	20g	8.5g	22g	11g	5.5g	1.9g

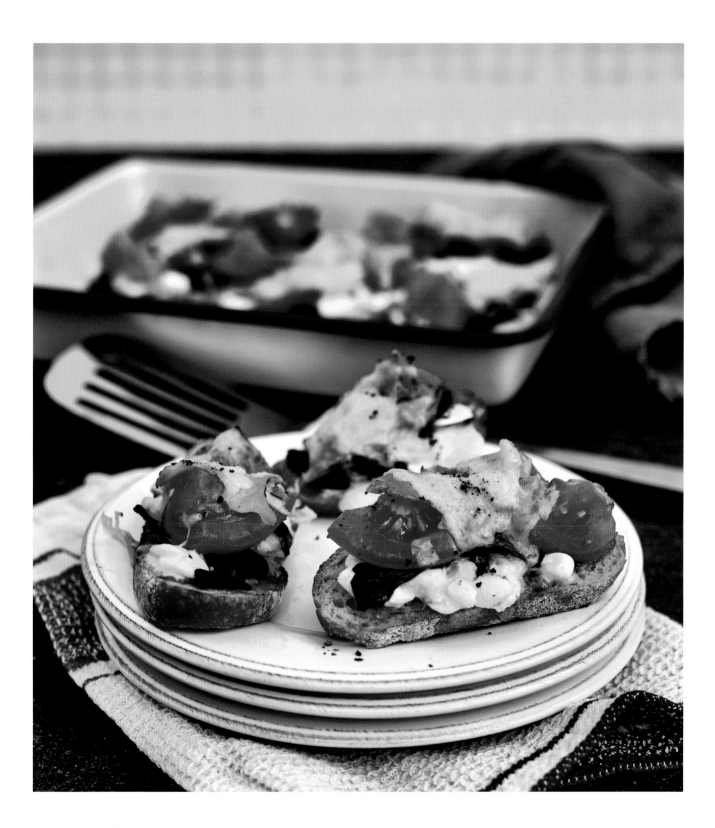

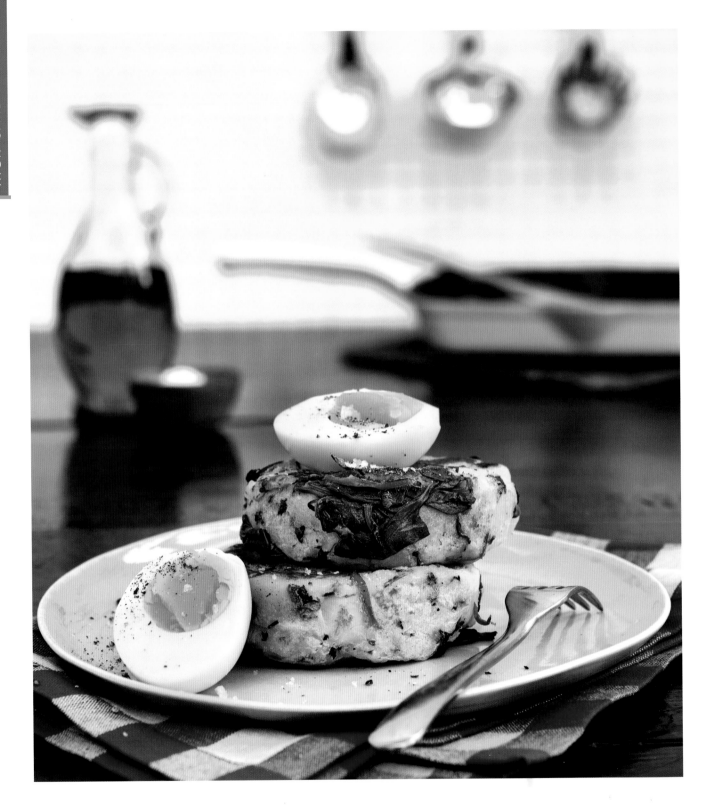

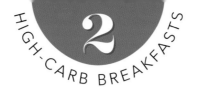

SPINACH, POTATO & CHILLI FRITTERS WITH BOILED EGGS

SERVES **2** ◆ PREP TIME **15 MINS** ◆ COOK TIME **25 MINS** ◆ DIFFICULTY **EASY** ◆ **GF** ◆ **DF** ◆ **V**

INGREDIENTS

3 medium potatoes, peeled and diced

2 handfuls baby spinach

1 small bunch coriander, finely chopped

1 hot red chilli, finely chopped

1 tablespoon olive oil

4 large eggs

OMAR SAYS: 'This dish is great served with the yoghurt hollandaise from the Eggs Royale, page 74.'

METHOD

1. Preheat your oven to 180°C.

2. Place the potatoes in a medium saucepan and cover with cold water. Bring to the boil and continue to cook over a medium heat for 10-15 minutes or until the potatoes are cooked through. Drain and allow to sit for 5 minutes.

3. Tip the potatoes into a large mixing bowl and gently crush together. Add the spinach and allow the heat from the potatoes to wilt the spinach. Mix in the coriander and chilli. Make the potatoes into 4 small burger shapes and chill in the fridge for 10 minutes.

4. Heat the olive oil in a frying pan over a medium heat. Carefully add the fritters one by one and cook on each side for 2 minutes or until golden brown. Divide between 2 plates.

5. Fill a saucepan with water and bring to the boil. Carefully add the eggs to the water and once the water is boiling again cook the eggs for 5 minutes. Run under cold water before peeling away the shell and slice into halves. Serve the eggs with the fritters.

PER SERVING

CARBS	ENERGY	FAT	SATURATES	PROTEIN	SUGAR	FIBRE	SALT
56g	500 kcal	18.5g	4.5g	24g	2.5g	6g	0.6g

6 69014 44890 3

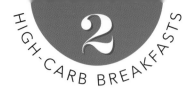
EGGS ROYALE WITH YOGHURT HOLLANDAISE

SERVES **2** ◆ PREP TIME **10 MINS** ◆ COOK TIME **5 MINS** ◆ DIFFICULTY **EASY**

INGREDIENTS
2 English muffins
4 slices smoked salmon
2 small handfuls watercress
2 teaspoons white wine vinegar
4 large eggs

YOGHURT HOLLANDAISE SAUCE
4 tablespoons Greek yoghurt
Juice of 1 lemon
1 teaspoon Dijon mustard
½ teaspoon Tabasco sauce

OMAR SAYS: 'Yoghurt hollandaise is an easy, no-cook take on the traditional sauce.'

METHOD
1. In a bowl whisk together the ingredients for the yoghurt hollandaise sauce then set aside.

2. Preheat your grill to high. Slice the muffins in half and toast under the grill. Place all the muffins on an oven tray and top each half with a slice of smoked salmon then the watercress.

3. Half-fill a small saucepan with water and bring to the boil. Turn down to a simmer and add the vinegar. Gently crack the eggs into the water and cook for 3 minutes. Drain and place an egg on top of each muffin half.

4. Spoon the hollandaise sauce over each egg and pop the tray under the grill for 30 seconds. Divide between two plates and serve.

PER SERVING

CARBS	ENERGY	FAT	SATURATES	PROTEIN	SUGAR	FIBRE	SALT
33g	484kcal	21g	6.5g	33g	4g	2.5g	2.8g

6 69014 44891 0

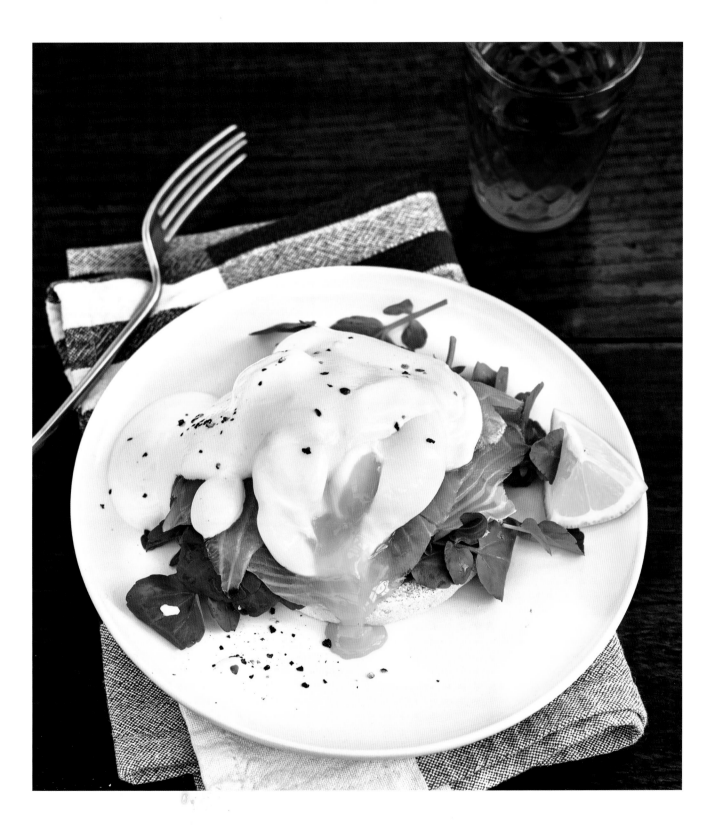

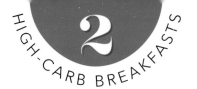

BIRCHER MUESLI

SERVES **4** ◆ PREP TIME **10 MINS** ◆ DIFFICULTY **EASY** ◆ **V**

INGREDIENTS

300g porridge oats
1 teaspoon ground cinnamon
1 pinch ground nutmeg
2 tablespoons demerara sugar
2 tablespoons sultanas
1 apple, cored and chopped
1 orange, peeled and chopped
500ml milk
3 tablespoons Greek yoghurt

OMAR SAYS: 'You can add your choice of fresh fruit, nuts, seeds or coconut. Serve with fresh apple slices and grated fresh ginger for an extra zing.'

METHOD

1. Mix together all the dry ingredients and the dried and fresh fruit in a large bowl. Pour over the milk and yoghurt and give it a good stir. Cover the bowl and place in the fridge overnight.

2. Next day, remove from the fridge and decorate with your choice of fresh fruit, grated orange peel or grated fresh ginger, if liked.

PER SERVING

CARBS	ENERGY	FAT	SATURATES	PROTEIN	SUGAR	FIBRE	SALT
68g	451 kcal	12g	5g	14g	24g	7.5g	0.15g

6 69014 44892 7

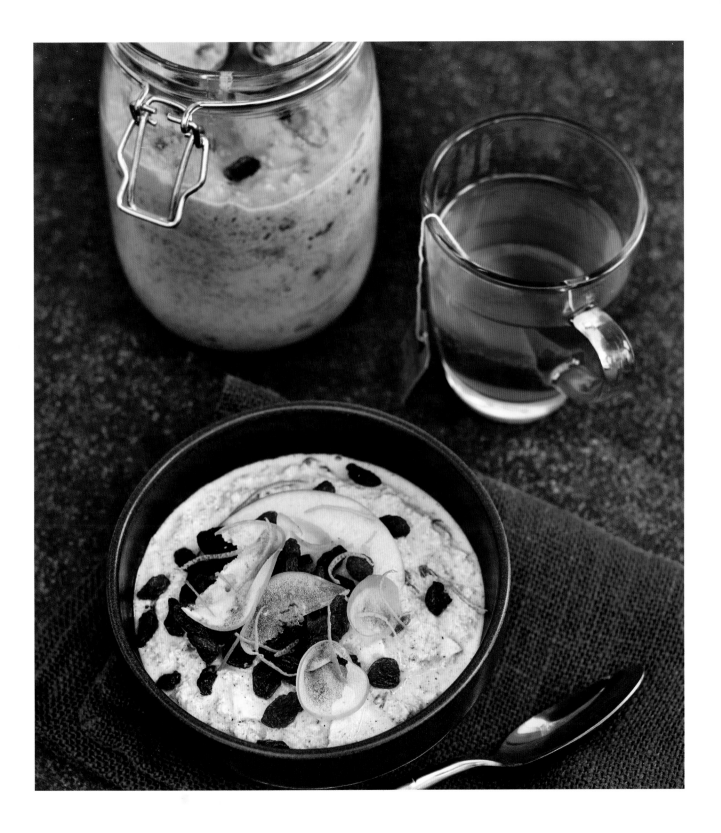

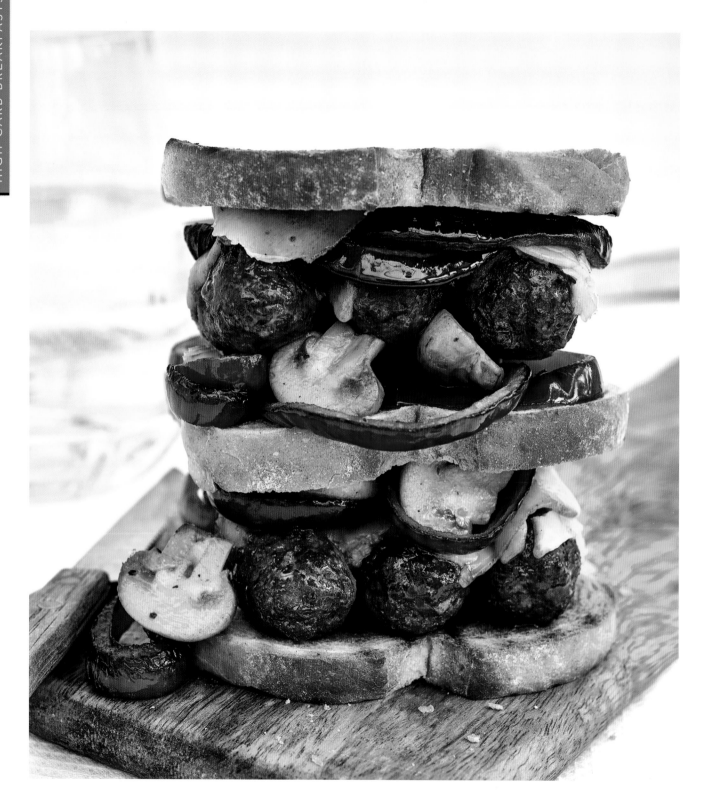

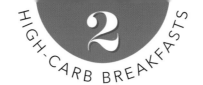

HOMEMADE BEEF SAUSAGE SANDWICH

SERVES **2** ◆ PREP TIME **10 MINS** ◆ COOK TIME **20 MINS** ◆ DIFFICULTY **EASY**

INGREDIENTS

300g minced beef
1 teaspoon ground cumin
2-3 knobs of butter
1 red onion, finely sliced
8 button mushrooms, roughly sliced
4 slices sourdough bread
50g smoked Cheddar, sliced

JAMES SAYS: 'White sourdough tastes great, but for healthier, complex carbs use wholemeal bread instead.'

METHOD

1. Preheat your oven to 180°C.

2. In a mixing bowl combine the minced beef and cumin and season with salt and pepper. Shape into 6 small sausages and chill in the fridge for 30 minutes.

3. Melt the butter in a frying pan over a medium heat. Add the onion to the pan and cook for 5 minutes. Next add the mushrooms. Season with salt and pepper and cook for a further 5 minutes, stirring continuously. Set the pan aside and keep warm.

4. Place the sausages on a roasting tray and bake in the oven for 10 minutes or until cooked through. Allow to rest for 5 minutes.

5. Toast the sourdough bread. Slice the sausages lengthways and divide between 2 slices of the toast. Top the sausage with the sliced Cheddar. Top the Cheddar with the mushrooms and onion. Top with the remaining slices of toast and serve.

PER SERVING

CARBS	ENERGY	FAT	SATURATES	PROTEIN	SUGAR	FIBRE	SALT
42g	709 kcal	39g	18.5g	45g	7g	4g	1.65g

6 69014 44893 4

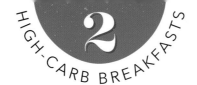

LEFT-OVER CHICKEN KEDGEREE

SERVES **4** ◆ PREP TIME **10 MINS** ◆ COOK TIME **35 MINS** ◆ DIFFICULTY **EASY** ◆ **GF** ◆ **DF**

INGREDIENTS

1 tablespoon olive oil
½ onion, finely chopped
1 garlic clove, finely chopped
2 tablespoons medium curry powder
250g basmati rice
1 litre water
200g cooked leftover chicken, chopped
1 small bunch coriander, chopped
1 handful baby spinach
150g frozen peas
4 large eggs

OMAR SAYS: 'This is even quicker with leftover or pre-cooked rice instead. Add it to the pan with just a splash of water and heat thoroughly.'

METHOD

1. Heat the olive oil in a large saucepan over a medium heat. Add the onion and garlic to the pan and cook without colouring for 2 minutes. Stir in the curry powder and then the rice. Mix everything together well. Pour over the water and add a good pinch of salt. Bring the pan to the boil and then turn down to a simmer and cook for 20 minutes or until the rice is cooked through and the water has been absorbed.
2. Stir the chicken and coriander into the rice, along with the spinach and peas. Give this a good mix. Place a lid on the pan and leave to one side for 5 minutes.
3. Meanwhile, half-fill a small saucepan with water and bring to the boil. Carefully add the eggs to the water and cook for 5 minutes. Run under cold water before peeling away the shells. Slice the eggs in half.
4. Divide the kedgeree between 4 plates and top with the soft-boiled eggs. Sprinkle with pepper and serve.

PER SERVING

CARBS	ENERGY	FAT	SATURATES	PROTEIN	SUGAR	FIBRE	SALT
57g	484 kcal	12.5g	3g	33g	2g	5.5g	0.45g

6 69014 44894 1

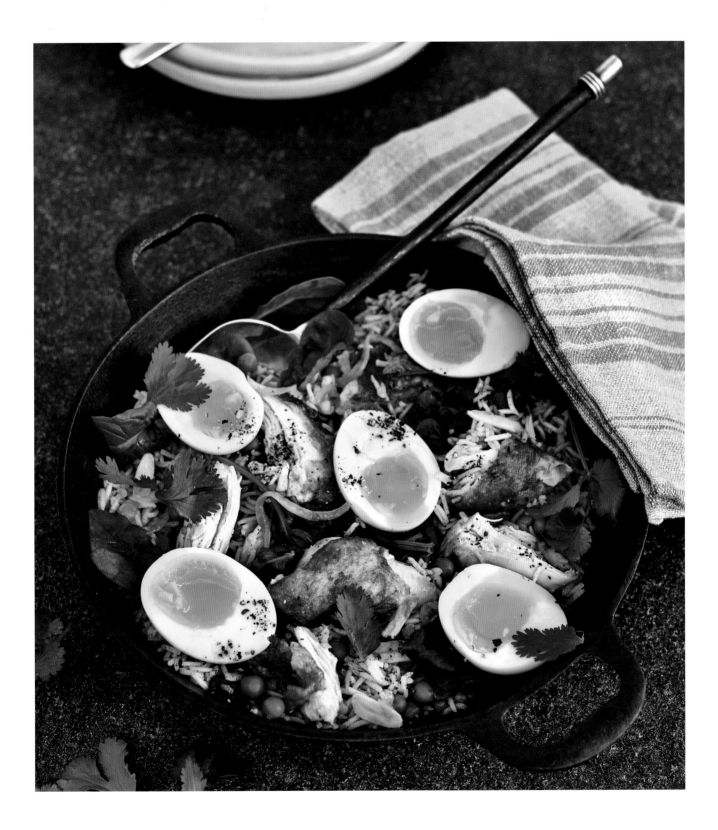

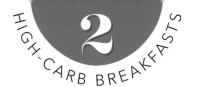

OVERNIGHT CHIA

PASSION FRUIT, COCONUT & ALMOND

SERVES **2** ◆ PREP TIME **10 MINS** ◆ DIFFICULTY **EASY** ◆ **GF** ◆ **DF** ◆ **V**

INGREDIENTS
40g chia seeds
240ml half-fat coconut milk
1 passion fruit
1 teaspoon desiccated coconut
1 teaspoon flaked almonds
2 teaspoons honey

METHOD
1. Place the chia seeds in a medium-sized bowl, pour over the coconut milk and whisk well. Pour the chia mixture into two serving cups or jars and place in the fridge overnight, or for at least 3 hours.

2. The next morning, slice the passion fruit in half and scoop out the seeds onto the top of the chia puddings. Sprinkle over the desiccated coconut and flaked almonds, drizzle over the honey and serve.

PER SERVING

CARBS	ENERGY	FAT	SATURATES	PROTEIN	SUGAR	FIBRE	SALT
17.5g	274 kcal	18.5g	10g	5g	8g	8.5g	Trace

PEANUT BUTTER & BANANA

SERVES **2** ◆ PREP TIME **5 MINS** ◆ DIFFICULTY **EASY** ◆ **GF** ◆ **DF** ◆ **V**

INGREDIENTS
40g chia seeds
240ml almond milk
1 tablespoon Meridian Peanut Butter
1 banana
1 teaspoon honey

METHOD
1. Place the chia seeds in a medium-sized bowl, pour over the almond milk and whisk well. Pour the chia mixture into two serving cups or jars and place in the fridge overnight, or for at least 3 hours.

2. The next morning, spoon the peanut butter over the chia puddings. Peel and slice the banana and add to the top of the chia puddings. Drizzle over the honey and serve.

PER SERVING

CARBS	ENERGY	FAT	SATURATES	PROTEIN	SUGAR	FIBRE	SALT
25.5g	246 kcal	11g	1.5g	6.5g	15.5g	9g	0.16g

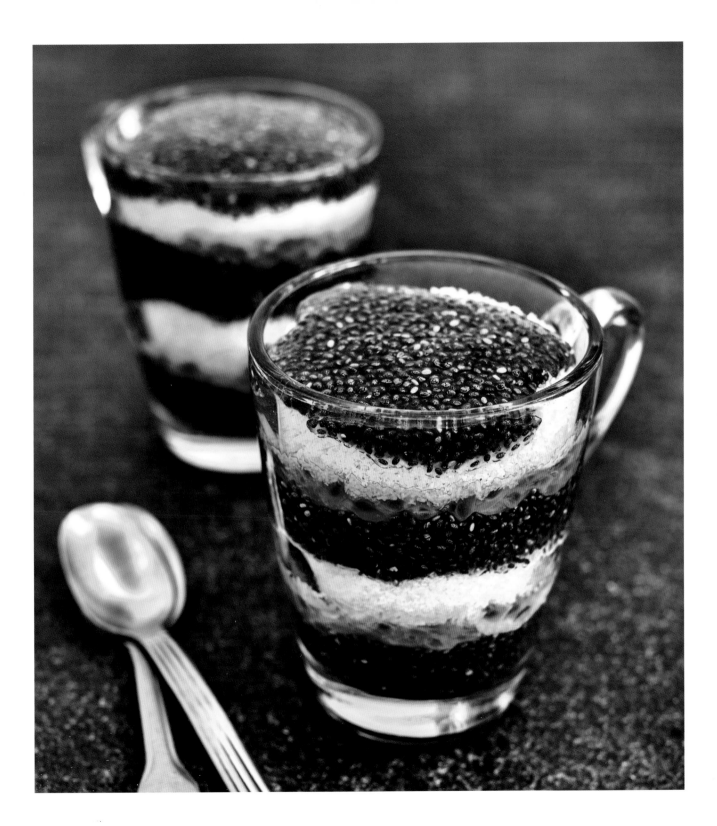

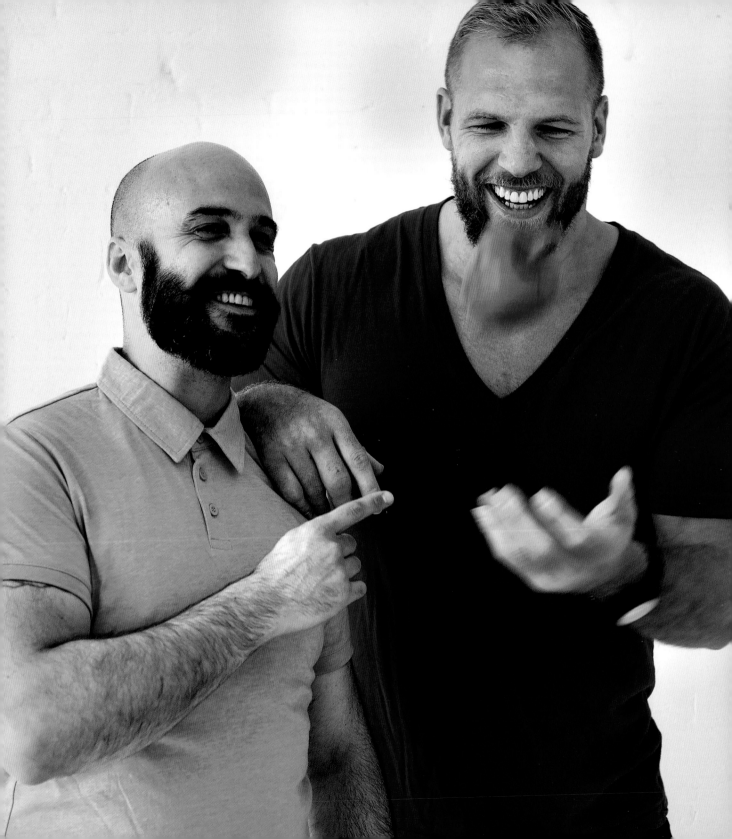

3

LOW-CARB LUNCHES

These recipes are predominantly made up of lean protein and non-starchy veg. Perfect for rest days when I'm trying to reduce my body fat percentage at the start of the season.

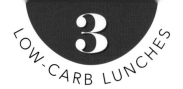

TRICOLORE SALAD

SERVES **2** ◆ PREP TIME **15 MINS** ◆ DIFFICULTY **EASY** ◆ **GF** ◆ **V**

INGREDIENTS

1 tablespoon hazelnuts
1 tablespoon almonds
2 beef tomatoes, or any other tomato variety will do
1 punnet cherry tomatoes
8-10 basil leaves
1 ball mozzarella
1 avocado, peeled and chopped
1 tablespoon pumpkin seeds
2 tablespoons olive oil
1 tablespoon balsamic vinegar

JAMES SAYS: 'The nuts and seeds are an excellent source of vitamins and minerals.'

METHOD

1. Crush the hazelnuts and almonds with a knife.
2. Remove the core from the beef tomatoes and chop into chunks or quarters. Slice the cherry tomatoes in half then place all the tomatoes in a mixing bowl.
3. Roughly tear the basil leaves and mix them in with the tomatoes. Tear the mozzarella into pieces then add them as well. Add the avocado, nuts and pumpkin seeds to the tomatoes. Drizzle over the olive oil and balsamic vinegar. Season with salt and pepper and give the salad a good toss . Divide between 2 plates and serve.

PER SERVING

CARBS	ENERGY	FAT	SATURATES	PROTEIN	SUGAR	FIBRE	SALT
11g	600 kcal	51g	14.5g	20g	9g	7g	0.65g

6 69014 44897 2

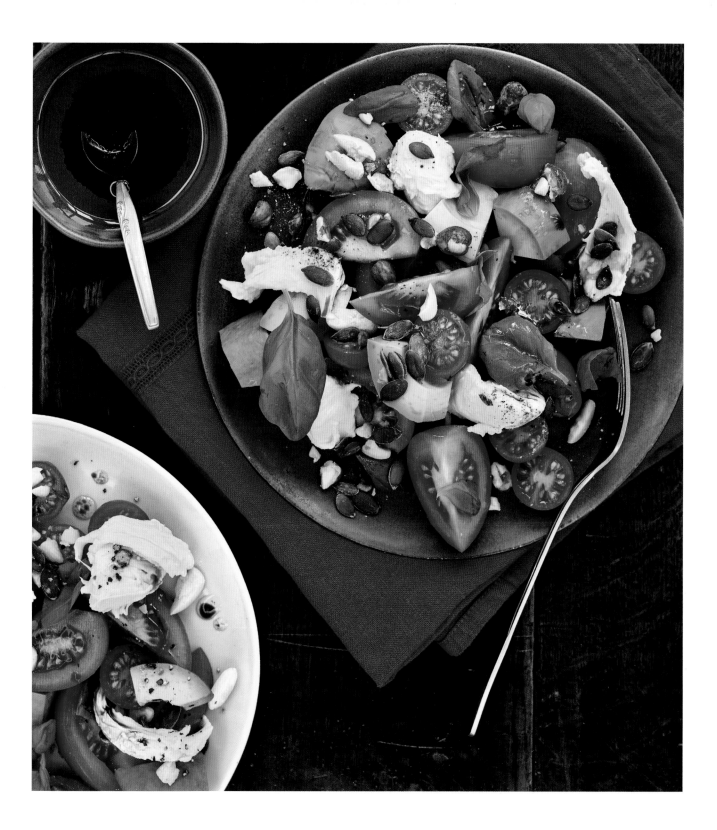

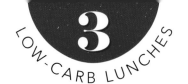

SPINACH, GINGER & CHILLI BALLS WITH THAI MANGO SALAD

SERVES **2** ◆ PREP TIME **20 MINS** ◆ COOK TIME **15 MINS** ◆ DIFFICULTY **EASY** ◆ **GF** ◆ **DF** ◆ **VG**

INGREDIENTS

SPINACH BALLS
1 handful baby spinach
½ red chilli
1 garlic clove
½ small bunch coriander
1 tablespoon olive oil
1 tablespoon medium curry powder
200g tinned butter beans

MANGO SALAD
1 mango, peeled and cubed
½ red chilli, finely chopped
1 garlic clove, finely chopped
1 red onion, finely sliced
1 carrot, grated
10 mangetouts
¼ cucumber, cut into fine batons

METHOD

1. Preheat your oven to 200°C

2. To make the spinach balls, place the spinach, chilli, garlic and coriander in a food processor and blend until it is all finely chopped. Now add the olive oil, curry powder and butter beans and pulse until it comes together to form a rough paste. Season with salt and pepper. Roll into 12 balls and put in the fridge for 30 minutes to firm up. Now place the balls on a lined baking tray and bake in the oven for 10-12 minutes.

3. Place the mango in a mixing bowl with the chilli and garlic. Add the red onion, carrot, mangetouts and the cucumber. Give it a good toss and divide between 2 serving bowls. Top the salad with the spinach balls and serve.

PER SERVING

CARBS	ENERGY	FAT	SATURATES	PROTEIN	SUGAR	FIBRE	SALT
35g	280 kcal	8g	1g	10g	20g	16g	0.2g

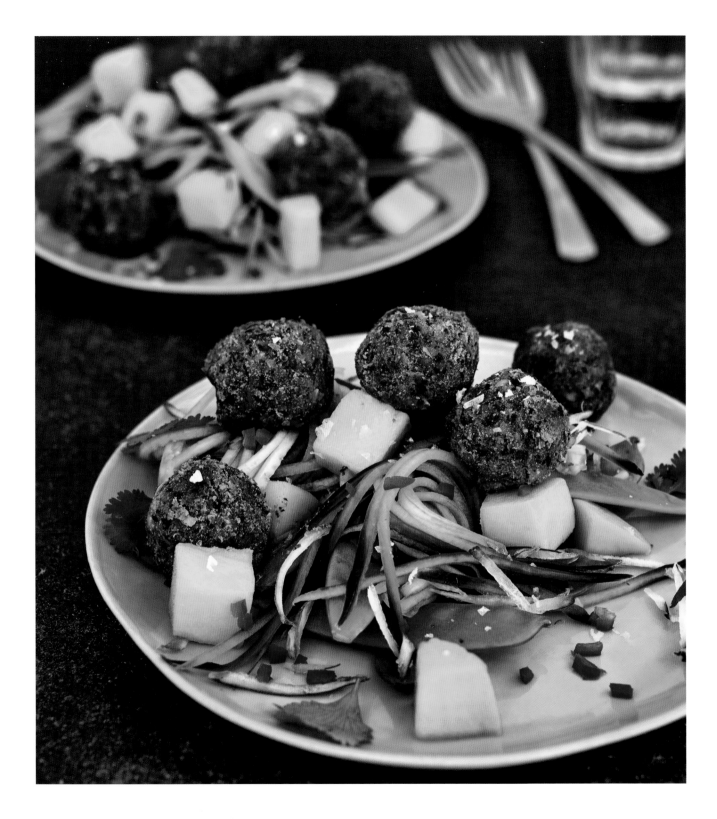

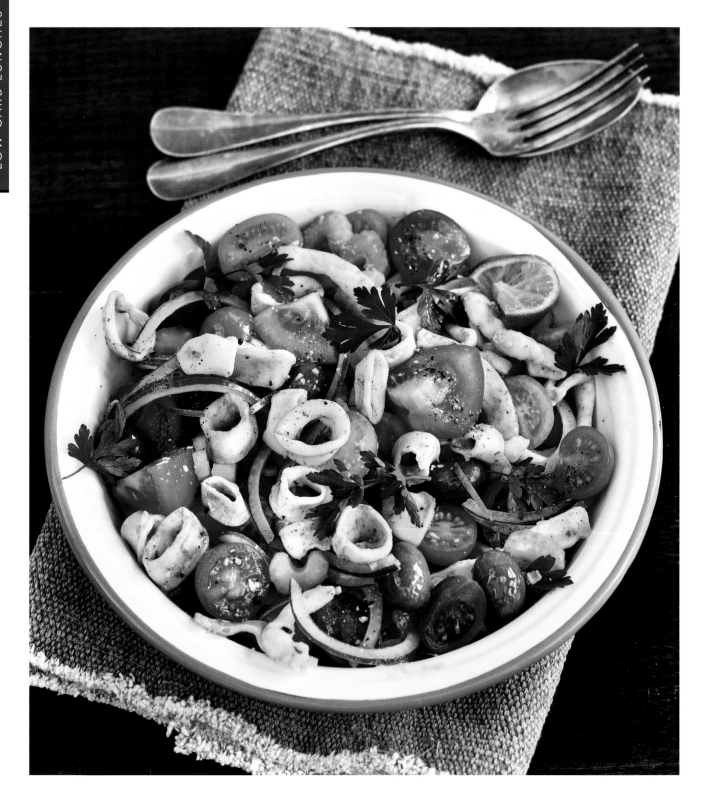

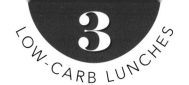
SPICY SQUID WITH BLOODY MARY TOMATO SALAD

SERVES **2** ◆ PREP TIME **10 MINS** ◆ COOK TIME **5 MINS** ◆ DIFFICULTY **EASY** ◆ **DF**

INGREDIENTS

300g raw squid rings
2 teaspoons Cajun seasoning
1 tablespoon olive oil
Juice of 1 lime, plus wedges to serve

TOMATO SALAD

1 red onion, finely sliced
1 punnet cherry tomatoes, halved
1 beef tomato, chopped into chunks
1 stick celery, finely chopped
2 tablespoons green olives, roughly chopped
½ teaspoon horseradish sauce
2 teaspoons Tabasco sauce
1 tablespoon white wine vinegar
1 tablespoon Worcestershire sauce

METHOD

1. Preheat your oven to 200°C.

2. Place the squid in a bowl and rub in the Cajun seasoning. Heat the olive oil in a frying pan over a high heat. Now add the squid and cook for 1-2 minutes. Transfer to a bowl and squeeze over the lime juice.

3. Place the red onion, cherry tomatoes and beef tomato in a mixing bowl. Mix in the celery and the olives. Add the horseradish, Tabasco sauce, vinegar and Worcestershire sauce, and season with salt and pepper. Give the salad a good toss and divide between two plates. Top the salad with the squid and a wedge of lime and serve.

PER SERVING

CARBS	ENERGY	FAT	SATURATES	PROTEIN	SUGAR	FIBRE	SALT
15g	273 kcal	11g	2g	26g	12g	5.5g	2.3g

6 69014 44899 6

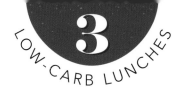

TURKEY WITH BEETROOT & STILTON SALAD

SERVES **2** ◆ PREP TIME **10 MINS** ◆ COOK TIME **12 MINS** ◆ DIFFICULTY **EASY** ◆ **GF**

INGREDIENTS
2 x 175g turkey escalopes
1 tablespoon olive oil
250g cooked beetroot
2 tablespoons walnut halves, roughly chopped
80g Stilton cheese
1 tablespoon balsamic vinegar
1 handful rocket leaves

METHOD
1. Preheat your grill to high.
2. Place the turkey escalopes on a tray and season with salt and pepper. Drizzle over the olive oil and grill for 5-6 minutes on each side until cooked through. Allow to rest for 5 minutes.
3. Cut the beetroots into quarters and place in a bowl. Add the walnuts and crumble the Stilton over the salad and drizzle over the vinegar. Give it a good toss to mix everything in.
4. Divide the rocket leaves between two plates and top with the beetroot salad. Slice the turkey and serve on top of the salad.

PER SERVING

CARBS	ENERGY	FAT	SATURATES	PROTEIN	SUGAR	FIBRE	SALT
13g	579kcal	32g	12g	58g	12.5g	4g	1.3g

6 69014 44900 9

MACKEREL WITH SWEET CHILLI SAUCE

SERVES **2** ◆ PREP TIME **5 MINS** ◆ COOK TIME **20 MINS** ◆ DIFFICULTY **EASY** ◆ **GF** ◆ **DF**

INGREDIENTS
2 red chillies, chopped
1 red pepper, chopped
1cm piece ginger, peeled and chopped
2 tablespoons Meridian Honey
100ml water
4 fillets fresh mackerel, about 100g each
1 tablespoon olive oil

METHOD
1. Place the chillies, red pepper, ginger, honey and water in a food processor and blend until smooth. Pour into a saucepan and heat over a low heat. Allow to simmer for 10-15 minutes. Remove from the heat and set aside.
2. Lay the mackerel on a plate skin-side down and season with salt and pepper, then leave the fish to sit for 5 minutes. Heat the olive oil in a frying pan over a medium heat. Gently lay the mackerel in the pan skin-side down. Cook the fish for 2 minutes before turning over and cooking for a further 1 minute. Spoon 2 tablespoons of chilli sauce over each mackerel fillet and remove from the heat.
3. Divide the mackerel between two plates and serve with salad of your choice, using the excess chilli sauce as a dressing.

PER SERVING

CARBS	ENERGY	FAT	SATURATES	PROTEIN	SUGAR	FIBRE	SALT
17g	605kcal	42g	9g	37g	20g	3.5g	0.9g

6 69014 44901 6

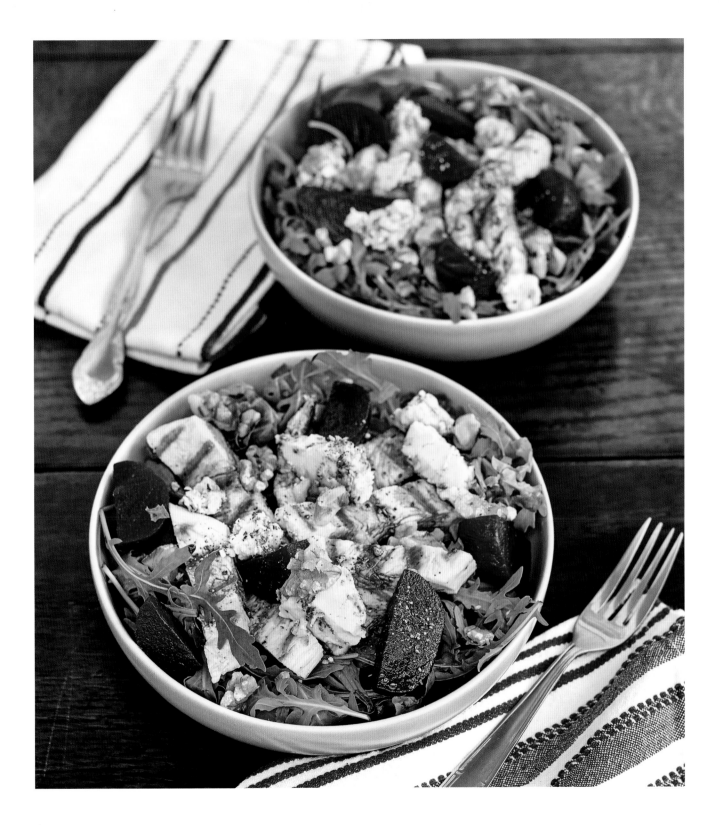

CHICKEN SHAWARMA SALAD BOWL

SERVES **2** ◆ PREP TIME **10 MINS** ◆ COOK TIME **20 MINS** ◆ DIFFICULTY **EASY** ◆ **GF** ◆ **DF**

INGREDIENTS

2 chicken breasts, skinless
2 garlic cloves, finely chopped
¼ red chilli, finely chopped
Zest and juice of 1 lemon
1 teaspoon ground cumin
1 teaspoon paprika
½ teaspoon turmeric
½ teaspoon ground cinnamon
8 radishes, sliced
10 cherry tomatoes, halved
½ red onion, finely sliced
¼ cucumber, sliced
2 spring onions, sliced
1 small bunch flat-leaf parsley, finely chopped

OMAR SAYS: 'Marinating the chicken in traditional Middle Eastern spices makes it succulent and delicious.'

METHOD

1. Preheat your oven to 200°C.

2. Mix together the chicken, garlic, chilli, lemon zest and juice in a large bowl. Add the cumin, paprika, turmeric and cinnamon to the chicken and mix well. Place in the fridge and leave for at least 1 hour to marinate. Now place the chicken on a roasting tray and bake in the oven for 15-20 minutes. Allow to rest for 5 minutes.

3. Place the radishes and cherry tomatoes in a mixing bowl. Add the red onion, cucumber and spring onions. Mix in the parsley, season with salt and pepper and toss well. Divide the salad between two plates, top with the chicken breasts and serve.

PER SERVING

CARBS	ENERGY	FAT	SATURATES	PROTEIN	SUGAR	FIBRE	SALT
5.5g	240kcal	7g	2g	38g	5g	1.5g	0.3g

6 69014 44902 3

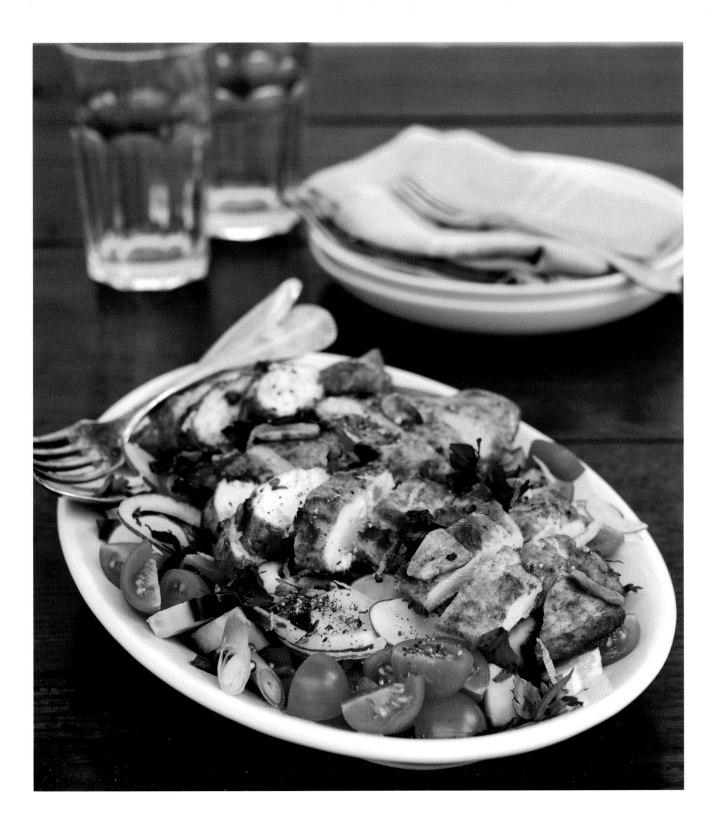

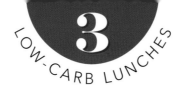

TOMATO & BUTTER BEAN SOUP WITH ROASTED COD

SERVES **2** ◆ PREP TIME **5 MINS** ◆ COOK TIME **40 MINS** ◆ DIFFICULTY **EASY** ◆ **GF** ◆ **DF**

INGREDIENTS

2 x 175g cod fillets

TOMATO SOUP
2 tablespoons olive oil
1 small carrot, chopped
1 stick celery, chopped
1 small onion, chopped
1kg tomatoes, chopped
2 garlic cloves, chopped
2 teaspoons tomato purée
1 teaspoon sugar
1 litre water
100g tinned butter beans

OMAR SAYS: 'The tomato soup can be prepared ahead up to the end of Step 2. Cool it then keep in the fridge for up to three days. Make sure it's piping hot before serving.'

METHOD

1. Preheat your oven to 200°C.

2. First make the tomato soup. Heat the olive oil in a large saucepan over a high heat. Add the carrot, celery and onion to the pan and cook for 2-3 minutes without colouring. Now add the tomatoes and garlic and cook for another 5 minutes. Add the tomato purée and sugar, and season with salt and pepper. Pour over the water, bring to the boil, then turn down to a simmer. Allow to cook for 25 minutes, before removing from the heat.

3. Allow the soup to cool for 10-15 minutes before blending until smooth in a food processor. Check the seasoning and then add the butter beans. Pour the soup back into the saucepan and warm over a low heat.

4. Place the cod fillets on a roasting tray and season with salt and pepper. Bake in the oven for 10 minutes or until cooked through.

5. Pour the soup into two bowls, place a fillet of cod into each bowl and serve.

PER SERVING

CARBS	ENERGY	FAT	SATURATES	PROTEIN	SUGAR	FIBRE	SALT
32g	418kcal	13g	2g	38g	23g	11g	0.5g

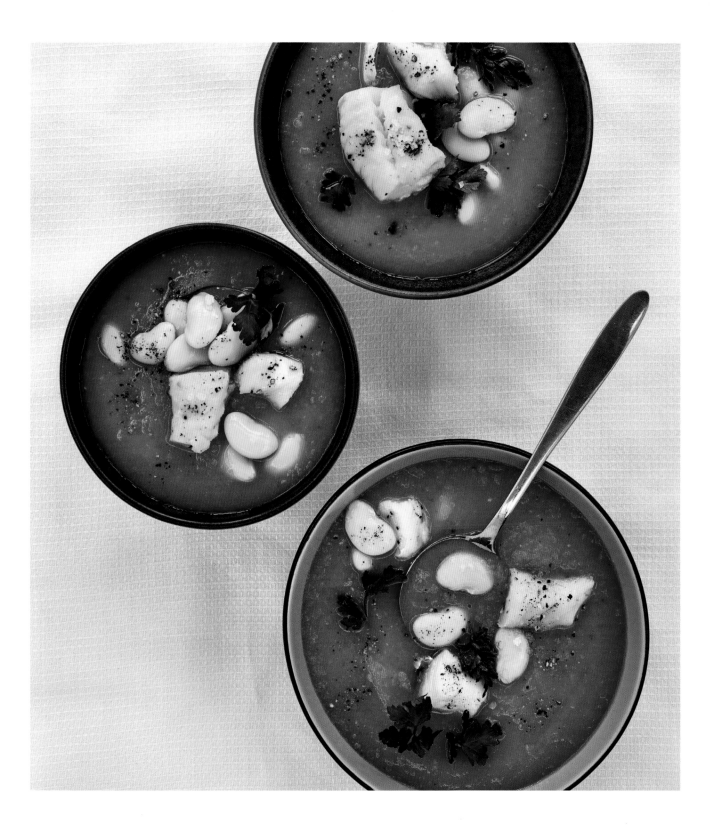

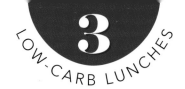

CURRIED CHICKEN & ROASTED CAULIFLOWER SALAD

SERVES **2** ◆ PREP TIME **15 MINS** ◆ COOK TIME **20 MINS** ◆ DIFFICULTY **EASY** ◆ **GF**

INGREDIENTS

1 tablespoon Greek yoghurt
1 tablespoon curry powder
2 chicken breasts

CAULIFLOWER SALAD

½ head of cauliflower, cut into florets
1 tablespoon olive oil
1 pinch ground cinnamon
1 pinch ground cumin
2 tablespoons hazelnuts, roughly chopped
1 small bunch flat-leaf parsley, chopped
1 pomegranate, halved
1 tablespoon white wine vinegar

METHOD

1. Preheat your oven to 180°C.

2. Combine the Greek yoghurt and curry powder in a large bowl. Coat the chicken breasts in the yoghurt and allow to marinate in the fridge for at least 30 minutes. Now place the chicken on a roasting tray and bake in the oven for 20 minutes or until the chicken is cooked through. Allow the chicken to rest for 10 minutes.

3. Place the cauliflower florets on a roasting tray. Drizzle over the olive oil and season with salt and pepper. Sprinkle over the cinnamon and cumin and give the cauliflower a good toss. Roast in the oven for 20 minutes or until the cauliflower has started to brown and is cooked through. Transfer to a large bowl. Add the hazelnuts and parsley to the cauliflower. Hold the pomegranate over the bowl and knock out the seeds with a wooden spoon. Now drizzle over the white wine vinegar and toss the salad.

4. Divide the salad between two plates. Slice the chicken breasts, place them on top of the salad and serve.

PER SERVING

CARBS	ENERGY	FAT	SATURATES	PROTEIN	SUGAR	FIBRE	SALT
19g	457 kcal	19g	3g	46g	13g	10g	0.4g

6 69014 44904 7

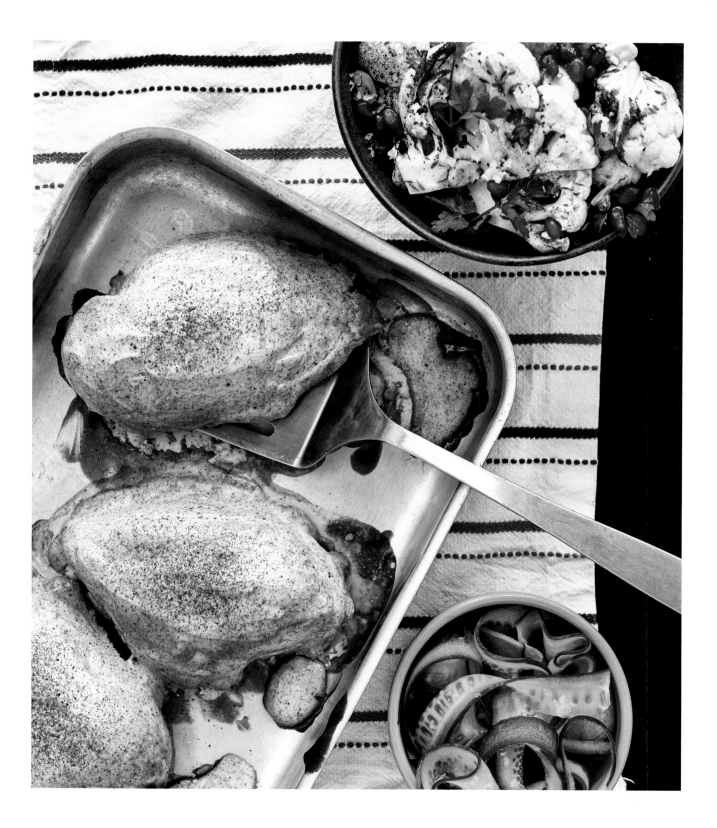

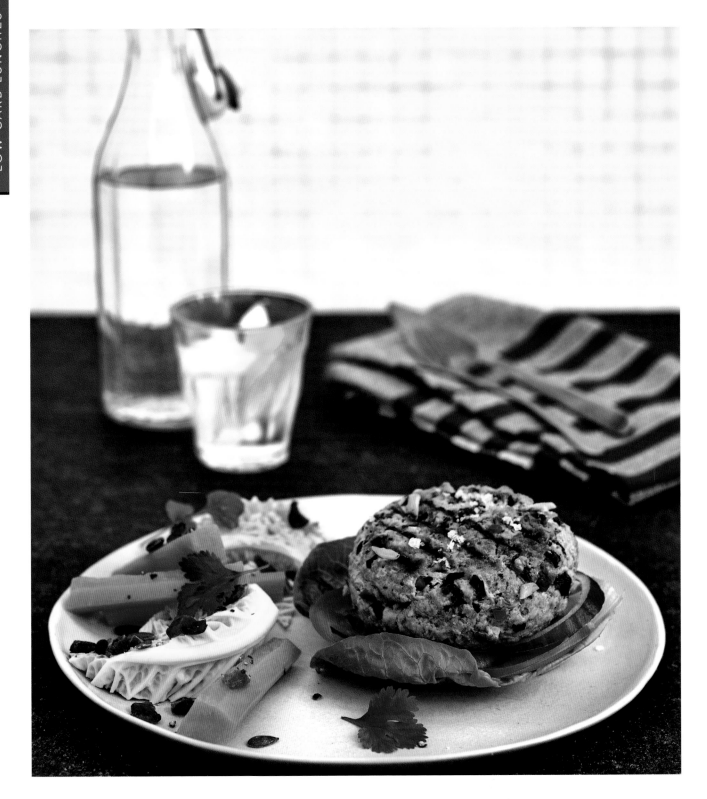

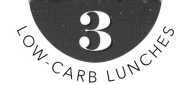
SKINNY LIME & CORIANDER PORK BURGER WITH CRUNCHY VEG SALAD

SERVES **2** ◆ PREP TIME **15 MINS** ◆ COOK TIME **25 MINS** ◆ DIFFICULTY **EASY** ◆ **GF** ◆ **DF**

INGREDIENTS

BURGERS

350g pork mince
Zest and juice of 1 lime
1 garlic clove, finely chopped
¼ red chilli, finely chopped
1 small bunch coriander, finely chopped

VEGETABLE SALAD

3 medium carrots, peeled and chopped into batons
½ red onion, finely chopped
1 wedge savoy cabbage (roughly ⅛ of a large cabbage), chopped
1 tablespoon dried cranberries
1 tablespoon pumpkin seeds
1 tablespoon sultanas
1 tablespoon white wine vinegar
½ teaspoon sugar

METHOD

1. Preheat your oven to 200°C.

2. Place the pork mince in a large bowl with the lime zest and juice, garlic, chilli and coriander. Mix together well and season with salt and pepper. Make into 2 burgers and place in the fridge for 30 minutes to firm up.

3. Place the burgers on a roasting tray and bake in the oven for 20 minutes or until cooked through. Allow to rest for 5 minutes.

4. Meanwhile, mix the carrots, onion and cabbage together in a large bowl. Sprinkle in the cranberries, pumpkin seeds and sultanas. Drizzle over the vinegar, add the sugar and give it a good toss. Divide the salad between two plates and top with the burgers.

PER SERVING

CARBS	ENERGY	FAT	SATURATES	PROTEIN	SUGAR	FIBRE	SALT
30.5g	495kcal	21.5g	7g	39g	27.5g	11g	0.5g

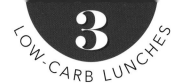

PRAWN LAKSA

SERVES **2** ◆ PREP TIME **15 MINS** ◆ COOK TIME **15 MINS** ◆ DIFFICULTY **EASY** ◆ **DF**

INGREDIENTS

2 courgettes
2 carrots, peeled
1 tablespoon coconut oil
200ml half-fat coconut milk
300ml water
Juice of 1 lime
½ teaspoon sugar
10 large prawns (head and shell removed)
1 small bunch coriander, chopped
2 boiled eggs

LAKSA PASTE
1 red chilli
3 garlic cloves
1cm piece of ginger
½ onion
1 stick of lemongrass
2 tablespoons Meridian Cashew Butter

OMAR SAYS: 'If you're short of time, use a vegetable peeler to slice the courgettes and carrots into ribbons instead.'

METHOD

1. Place the ingredients for the laksa paste in a food processor and blend until smooth.

2. Using a vegetable knife, slice the courgettes and carrots into long noodle-like strands and set aside.

3. Heat the coconut oil in a large saucepan over a high heat. Add the laksa paste and cook for 1 minute. Pour in the coconut milk and water, then add in the lime juice and sugar. Bring this to the boil and then immediately turn down to a gentle simmer. Now add the prawns, courgettes and carrots, and cook for 2-3 minutes. Sprinkle the coriander into the soup. Season with salt and pepper.

4. Slice the boiled eggs in half. Divide the soup between two bowls, top with the eggs and serve.

PER SERVING

CARBS	ENERGY	FAT	SATURATES	PROTEIN	SUGAR	FIBRE	SALT
19g	477kcal	28g	15g	33g	14.5g	7g	0.8g

6 69014 44906 1

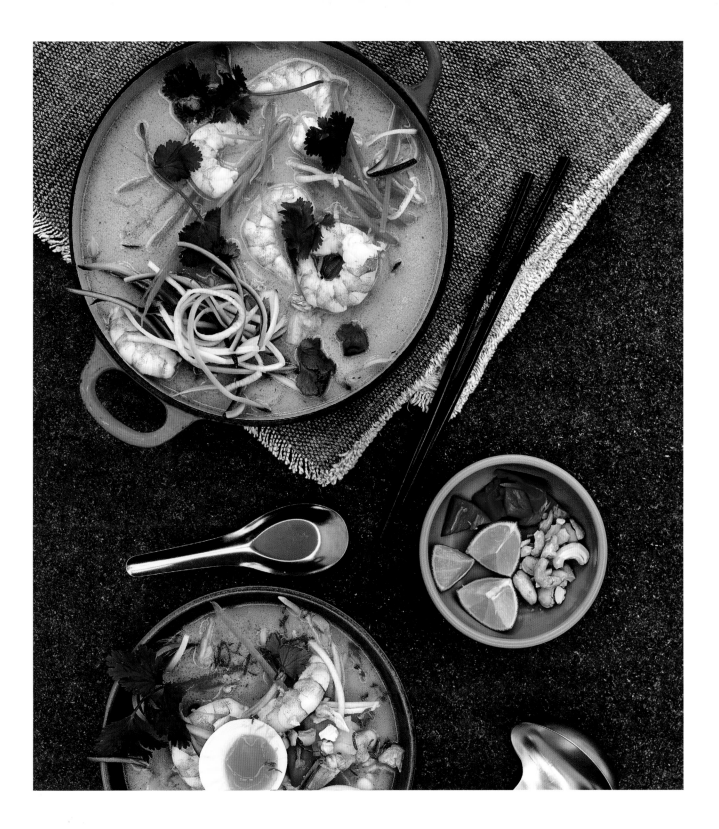

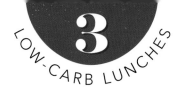
SMOKED SALMON FLATBREAD PIZZA

SERVES **4** ◆ PREP TIME **10 MINS** ◆ COOK TIME **15 MINS** ◆ DIFFICULTY **EASY**

INGREDIENTS

8 new potatoes
4 spring onions, finely sliced
½ red onion, finely sliced
1 small bunch dill, chopped
1 red chilli, chopped
200g smoked salmon, roughly chopped
4 small tortilla flat breads or small pitta breads, about 50g each
4 tablespoons cottage cheese
1 handful rocket leaves

JAMES SAYS: 'If you pre-cook and cool the potatoes, this is ready in less than 15 minutes.'

METHOD

1. Preheat your grill to medium.

2. Place the potatoes in a saucepan and cover with cold water. Bring to the boil on a high heat. Cook the potatoes for 10-12 minutes or until cooked through. Drain and run under cold water. When cool, cut each potato into quarters and place in a bowl. Mix the spring onions and red onion with the potatoes. Next stir in the dill, chilli and smoked salmon.

3. Lay the flatbreads out on the work surface and spread the cottage cheese over each one. Top with the salmon and potato mix. Place under the grill and cook for 2-3 minutes. Scatter over the rocket leaves, give a good grind of black pepper and serve.

PER SERVING

CARBS	ENERGY	FAT	SATURATES	PROTEIN	SUGAR	FIBRE	SALT
20g	340 kcal	8g	2g	20g	5g	8g	2g

6 69014 44907 8

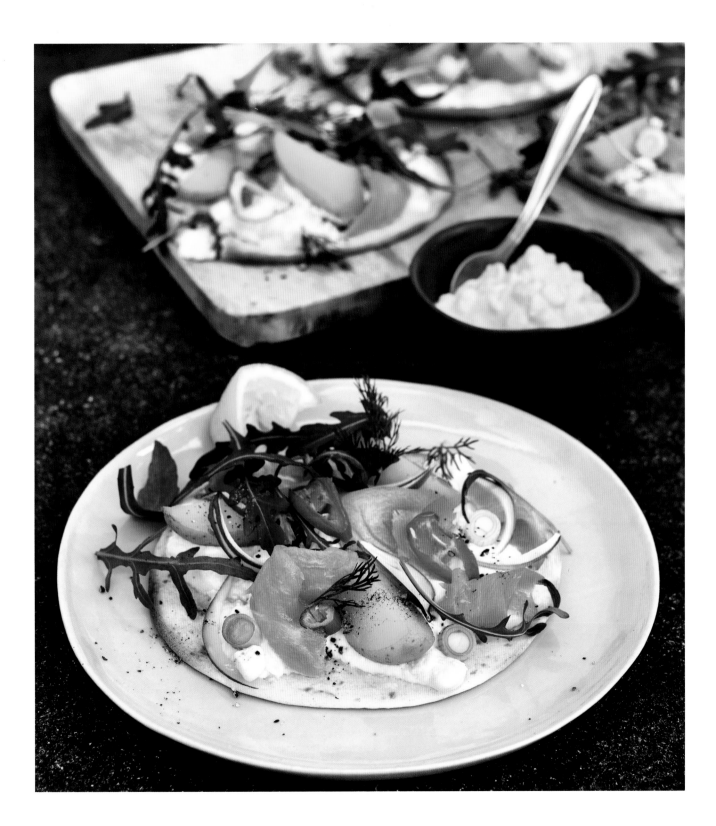

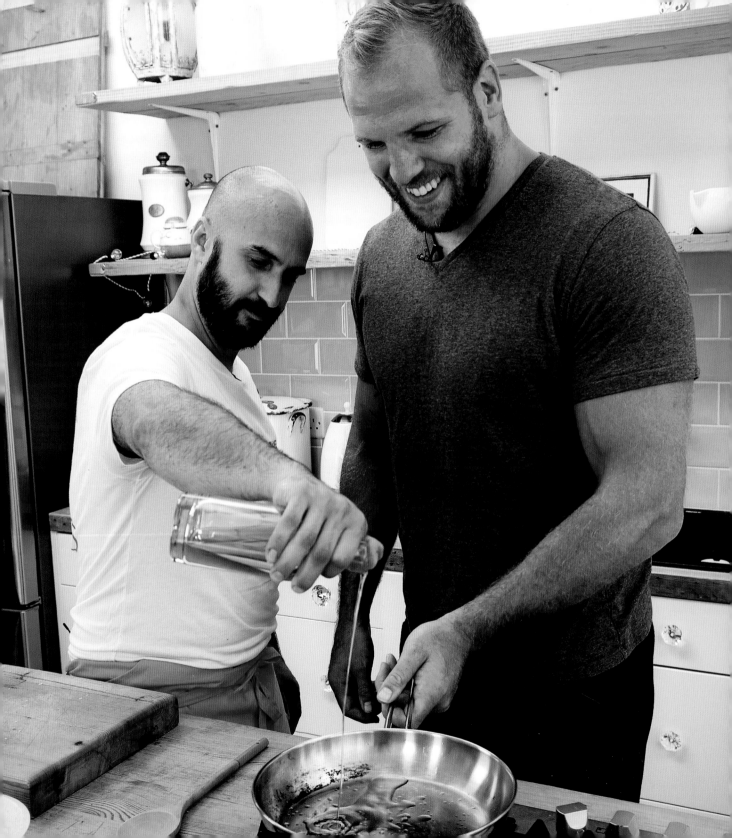

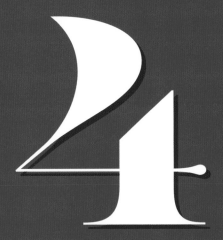

HIGH-CARB
LUNCHES

As a rugby player, I have to fuel my training and get the balance of my macros right. That means I have carbs, protein and fats in every meal throughout the day, albeit in the right quantities.

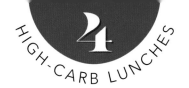

RAINBOW SALAD WITH SPICY RICE & TURKEY

SERVES **2** ◆ PREP TIME **5 MINS** ◆ COOK TIME **25 MINS** ◆ DIFFICULTY **EASY** ◆ **GF** ◆ **DF**

INGREDIENTS

180g brown rice
1 red chilli, finely sliced
1 garlic clove, finely sliced
50g tinned kidney beans, drained
100g edamame beans
2 x 175g turkey escalopes
1 tablespoon olive oil
6-8 cooked baby beetroots, quartered
2 carrots, peeled and grated
½ small bunch mint, roughly chopped

JAMES SAYS: 'I often have this after training as it has good amounts of carbs and protein.'

METHOD

1. Preheat your grill to high.

2. Place the rice in a saucepan and cover with water. Bring to the boil and cook over a high heat for 10-15 minutes or according to the pack instructions, until cooked. Drain and run under cold running water to stop the cooking process. Drain the rice again and place in a mixing bowl. Stir the chilli and garlic into the rice along with the kidney beans. Divide the rice between two serving plates and set aside.

3. Half-fill a small saucepan with water and bring to the boil, add the edamame beans and cook for 5 minutes. Drain and set aside.

4. Place the turkey escalopes on a roasting tray and season with salt and pepper. Drizzle over the olive oil and grill for 3-4 minutes on each side or until cooked through. Once the turkey is cooked allow it to rest for 5 minutes.

5. Mix together the beetroots, carrots, edamame beans and mint in a large bowl. Divide the salad between the two serving plates. Slice the turkey and serve on top of the salads.

PER SERVING

CARBS	ENERGY	FAT	SATURATES	PROTEIN	SUGAR	FIBRE	SALT
90g	742kcal	14.5g	3g	57g	15.5g	13g	0.62g

6 69014 44908 5

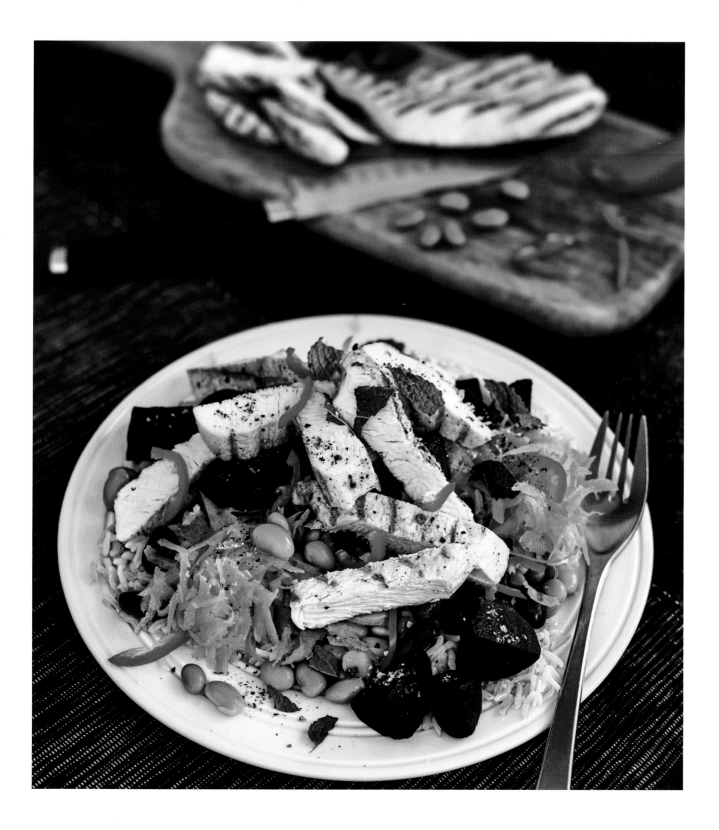

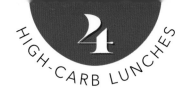

SPICY MEXICAN BEEF QUESADILLAS

SERVES **4** ◆ PREP TIME **10 MINS** ◆ COOK TIME **50 MINS** ◆ DIFFICULTY **EASY** ◆ **DF**

INGREDIENTS

1 tablespoon olive oil
400g lean beef mince
1 red chilli, finely chopped
2 teaspoons smoked paprika
1 teaspoon Cajun seasoning
1 tablespoon cocoa powder
200g tinned kidney beans, drained
400g tin chopped tomatoes
50g brown rice
2 tortilla wraps
1 baby gem lettuce, finely sliced
1 avocado, peeled and sliced

OMAR SAYS: 'Serve with a large salad of colourful leaves, peppers and tomatoes.'

METHOD

1. Preheat your oven to 180°C.

2. Heat the olive oil in a large saucepan over a high heat. Carefully add the beef mince and cook for 5 minutes or until the meat is browned well. Now add the chilli to the beef. Season with salt and pepper and add the paprika, Cajun spice and cocoa powder. Mix in the kidney beans and cook for another 2-3 minutes. Now add the chopped tomatoes and turn the heat down to a gentle simmer. Cook the beef for a further 20-25 minutes, stirring occasionally.

3. Place the rice in a saucepan and cover with water. Bring to the boil and cook the rice over a high heat for 10-15 minutes or according to the pack instructions. Once the rice is cooked, drain and set aside.

4. To arrange the quesadillas, lay one of the tortilla wraps out on a flat baking tray. Spoon the rice over the tortilla and then top with the beef chilli. Place the lettuce and avocado over the beef and top with the remaining tortilla. Bake in the oven for 10 minutes before serving.

PER SERVING

CARBS	ENERGY	FAT	SATURATES	PROTEIN	SUGAR	FIBRE	SALT
40g	471kcal	18g	5.5g	32.5g	5g	9.5g	1g

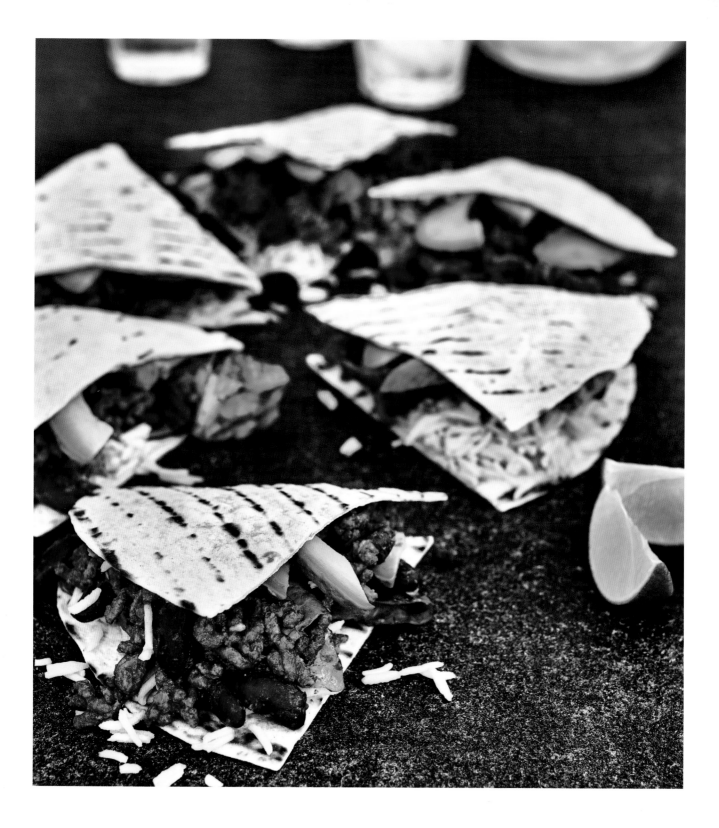

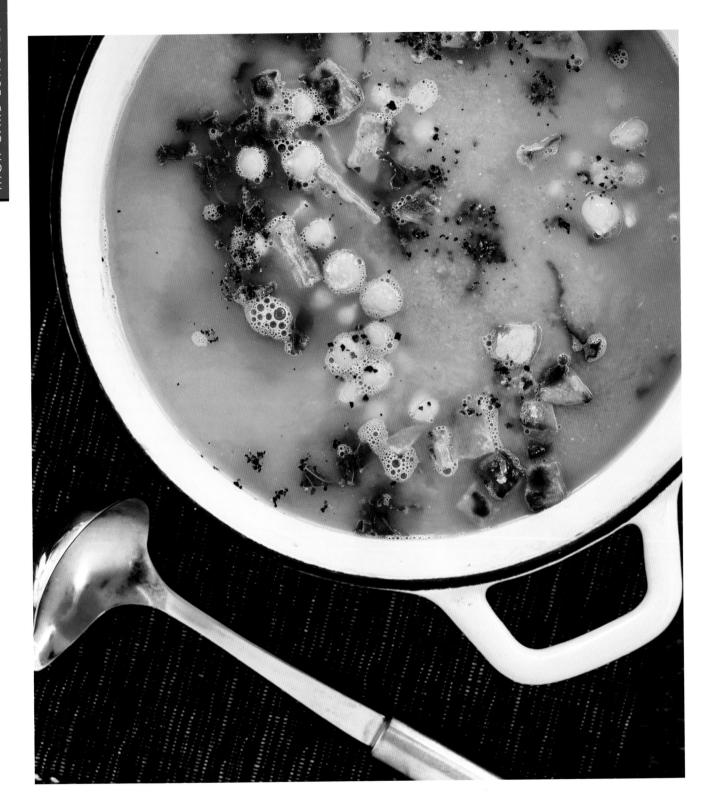

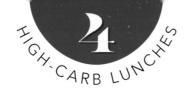

SWEET POTATO, CHICKPEA & KALE SOUP

SERVES **2** ◆ PREP TIME **5 MINS** ◆ COOK TIME **40 MINS** ◆ DIFFICULTY **EASY** ◆ **DF** ◆ **VG**

INGREDIENTS

1 tablespoon olive oil
1 garlic clove, finely sliced
1 large sweet potato, peeled and cut
into 2cm dice
400g tin chickpeas, drained
1.5 litres hot water
1 vegetable stock cube
1 pinch ground cinnamon
1 pinch ground cumin
4 large kale leaves, chopped

JAMES SAYS: 'I often make double as this soup keeps well in the fridge for a few days.'

METHOD

1. Preheat your oven to 200°C. Heat the olive oil in a large saucepan over a high heat. Place the garlic and half of the sweet potato in the pan and cook for 2-3 minutes without colouring. Add half of the chickpeas and continue to cook for 1 minute.

2. Boil the kettle and pour 1.5 litres of hot water into a jug, then dissolve the stock cube in the water. Pour the stock into the pan of sweet potato and add the cinnamon and cumin. Bring the soup to the boil and then turn down to a gentle simmer and cook for 25 minutes or until the sweet potato is cooked through. Allow the soup to cool a little before placing in a food processor and blending until smooth. Adjust the seasoning and pour back into the saucepan.

3. While the soup is cooking, place the remaining potato chunks on a baking tray and bake in the oven for 15-20 minutes or until cooked through.

4. Place the saucepan of soup over a low-medium heat and add the remaining chickpeas and the kale. Now add the baked sweet potato chunks into the soup. Serve as soon as the soup is nice and hot.

PER SERVING

CARBS	ENERGY	FAT	SATURATES	PROTEIN	SUGAR	FIBRE	SALT
60.5g	427kcal	11g	1.5g	13.5g	12g	15.4g	1.7g

6 69014 44910 8

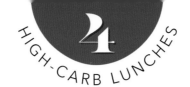

POSH MACKEREL FISH FINGER SANDWICHES

SERVES **2** ◆ PREP TIME **20 MINS** ◆ COOK TIME **5 MINS** ◆ DIFFICULTY **EASY** ◆ **DF**

INGREDIENTS

100g oats
2 eggs
50g plain flour
3 smoked mackerel fillets,
about 75g each
1 tablespoon olive oil
4 slices sourdough bread
4 baby gem lettuce leaves
2 tomatoes, sliced
2 boiled eggs, sliced

FOR THE SAUCE

1 tablespoon capers, finely chopped
2 gherkins, finely chopped
½ small bunch dill, finely chopped
2 tablespoons light mayonnaise
1 teaspoon Tabasco sauce
½ teaspoon smoked paprika

JAMES SAYS: 'This is high in fat and calories, so I'd have this as an occasional treat.'

METHOD

1. First make the sauce. Place the capers, gherkins and dill in a small bowl and stir in the mayonnaise, Tabasco sauce and smoked paprika. Set aside.
2. Pour the oats into a bowl. Whisk the eggs in another bowl. Pour the flour into another bowl. Now dip the mackerel into the flour, then into the egg and finally into the oats. Ensure that the fish picks up a good covering of the oats. Heat the olive oil in a frying pan over a low-medium heat. Carefully add the mackerel to the pan and cook for 2 minutes on each side or until the oats are golden brown.
3. Spread the sauce over each slice of the sourdough bread. Top two slices of the bread with the baby gem lettuce leaves and the tomato slices. Cut one of the mackerel pieces in half, then place one and a half pieces of fish on each slice, followed by the boiled egg slices. Top each one with the other slice of bread and serve.

PER SERVING

CARBS	ENERGY	FAT	SATURATES	PROTEIN	SUGAR	FIBRE	SALT
73g	970kcal	49g	9.5g	50g	7g	7.5g	3.25g

6 69014 44911 5

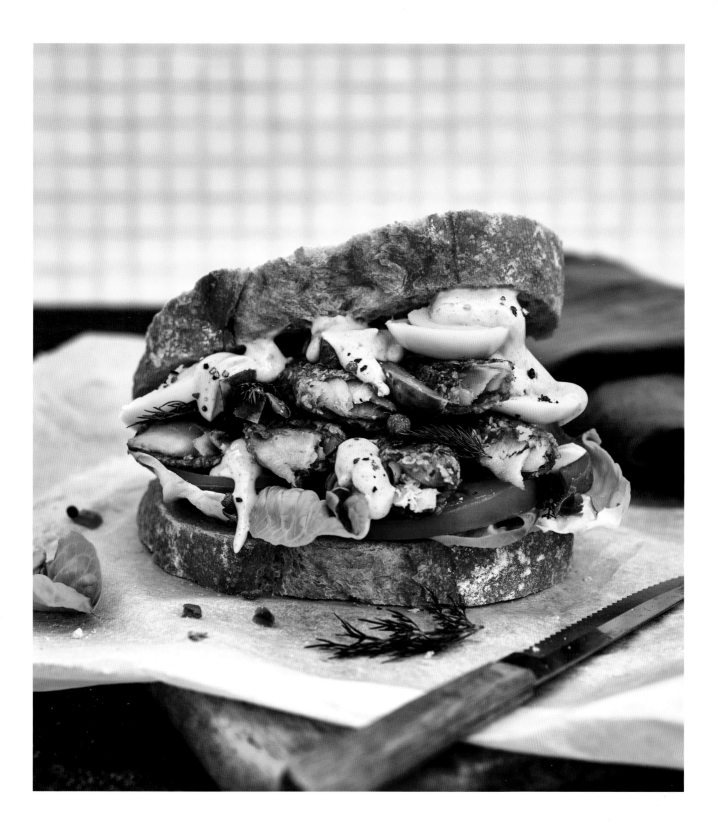

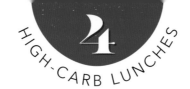

TURKEY, CHORIZO & PAPRIKA MEATBALLS WITH CHILLI POTATO SALAD

SERVES **2** ◆ PREP TIME **20 MINS** ◆ COOK TIME **30 MINS** ◆ DIFFICULTY **EASY** ◆ **DF**

INGREDIENTS

MEATBALLS
350g turkey mince
50g chorizo, finely chopped
1 garlic clove, finely chopped
1 teaspoon smoked paprika

POTATO SALAD
3-4 medium potatoes, peeled and cut into 2cm dice
50g green olives, roughly chopped
½ small bunch mint
2 spring onions, finely chopped
½ red chilli, finely chopped
½ red onion, finely chopped
1 tablespoon olive oil

DILL SAUCE
1 small bunch dill
Zest and juice of 1 lemon
1 garlic clove
2 tablespoons olive oil

METHOD

1. Preheat your oven to 180°C.

2. Mix together the turkey mince, chorizo, garlic and paprika in a large bowl. Season with salt and pepper. Shape into approximately 16 meatballs and pop them in the fridge for 30 minutes.

3. Place the potatoes in a saucepan and cover with cold water. Bring to the boil over a high heat and cook for 10 minutes or until cooked through. Drain and tip into a mixing bowl. Add the olives, mint, spring onions, red chilli and red onion and mix together with the potatoes. Drizzle over the olive oil and season with salt and pepper. Divide the potato salad between two plates.

4. Place the turkey balls on a roasting tray and bake them in the oven for 10-12 minutes or until cooked through. Remove from the oven and allow to rest for 5 minutes. Meanwhile, place the dill, lemon zest and juice, garlic and olive oil in a food processor and blend until smooth. Season with salt and pepper. Pour the sauce over the meatballs and give them a good mix. Divide the meatballs between the two plates and serve.

PER SERVING

CARBS	ENERGY	FAT	SATURATES	PROTEIN	SUGAR	FIBRE	SALT
60.5g	790 kcal	36g	8.5g	52g	6g	8g	2.2g

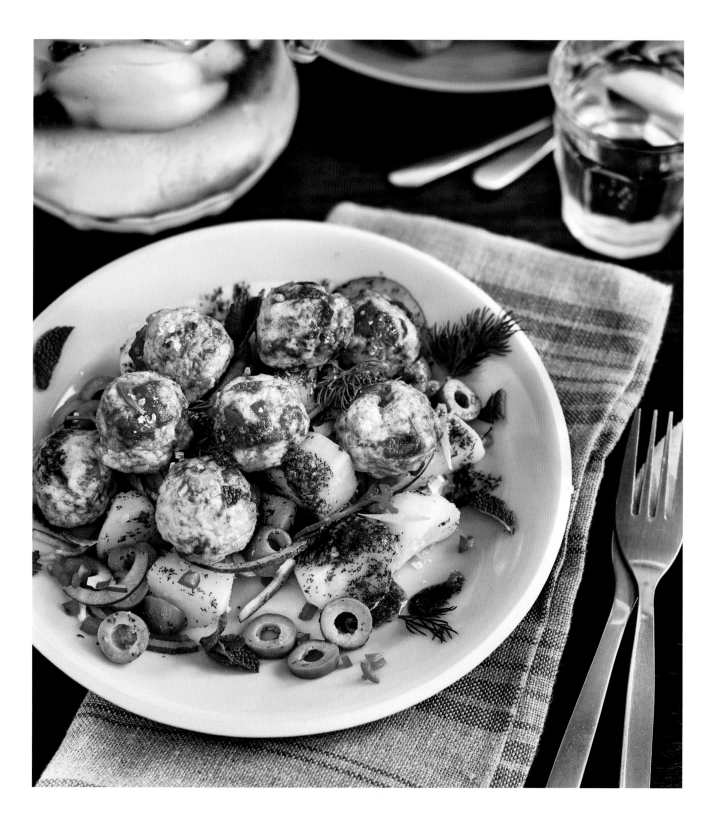

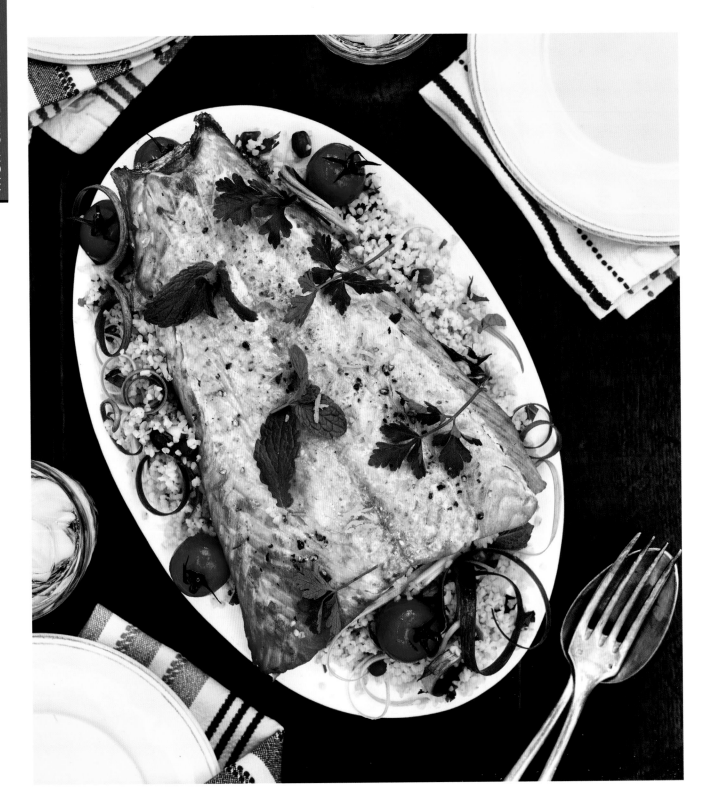

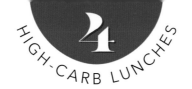

TABBOULEH SALAD WITH ROASTED SALMON

SERVES **2** ◆ PREP TIME **15 MINS** ◆ COOK TIME **10 MINS** ◆ DIFFICULTY **EASY** ◆ **DF**

INGREDIENTS

SALMON
2 salmon fillets
Juice of 1 lemon

TABBOULEH
80g bulgar wheat
1 bunch flat-leaf parsley, finely chopped
½ small bunch mint, finely chopped
4 tomatoes, diced
2 spring onions, finely chopped
1 pomegranate, halved
Zest and juice of 1 lemon
2 tablespoons olive oil

OMAR SAYS: 'Sprinkle lemon zest and sprigs of parsley over the salmon before serving.'

METHOD

1. Preheat your oven to 200°C.
2. First make the tabbouleh. In a colander wash the bulgar wheat until the water runs clear. Tip the bulgar wheat into a mixing bowl, boil the kettle and pour enough water over the wheat to just cover it. Cover the bowl with cling film and leave to one side for 30 minutes. Once the bulgar wheat is fluffy and cooked through, drain in a colander and pour back into the mixing bowl.
3. Mix the parsley and mint into the wheat. Stir in the tomatoes and spring onions. Hold the pomegranate over the bowl and knock the back with a wooden spoon until the seeds pop out and mix with the wheat. Add the lemon zest and juice, then drizzle over the olive oil and season with salt and pepper. Divide the tabbouleh between two plates.
4. Place the salmon on a roasting tray and season with salt and pepper. Bake in the oven for 8 minutes or until cooked through. Squeeze over the lemon juice and serve the salmon with the tabbouleh.

PER SERVING

CARBS	ENERGY	FAT	SATURATES	PROTEIN	SUGAR	FIBRE	SALT
45g	656kcal	35g	6g	37g	15g	9g	0.2g

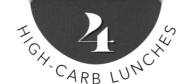

LAMB KEBABS WITH SPICY RICE & APPLE SLAW

SERVES **2** ◆ PREP TIME **20 MINS** ◆ COOK TIME **10 MINS** ◆ DIFFICULTY **EASY** ◆ **GF**

INGREDIENTS

LAMB KEBABS
400g lean lamb mince
2 garlic cloves, finely chopped
¼ red chilli, finely chopped
½ teaspoon ground cumin
½ teaspoon ground cinnamon
½ small bunch coriander, finely chopped

SPICY RICE
130g rice
1 teaspoon Cajun spice

APPLE SLAW
1 green apple, cored and grated
½ small white cabbage, finely shredded
1 carrot, peeled and grated
2 tablespoons Greek yoghurt
1 tablespoon mayonnaise

METHOD

1. Preheat your oven to 180°C.
2. Place the lamb mince in a large bowl and add the garlic, chilli, cumin, cinnamon and coriander. Mix well then divide into approximately 16 balls. Pop in the fridge for 30 minutes.
3. Meanwhile, pour the rice into a saucepan, cover with water and sprinkle in the Cajun spice. Bring to the boil and cook the rice for 10 minutes or according to the pack instructions until cooked through. Drain, cover and set aside.
4. Mix together the apple, cabbage and carrot in a bowl. Pour in the yoghurt and mayonnaise and give the coleslaw a good mix. Season with salt and pepper and divide between two serving plates.
5. Place the lamb kebabs on a roasting tray and bake in the oven for 8-10 minutes. Once cooked, allow them to rest for 5 minutes. Serve the lamb kebabs with the spicy rice and the apple slaw, with lemon wedges to squeeze over, if liked.

PER SERVING

CARBS	ENERGY	FAT	SATURATES	PROTEIN	SUGAR	FIBRE	SALT
65g	711kcal	28g	12g	48g	12.5g	6g	1g

6 69014 44914 6

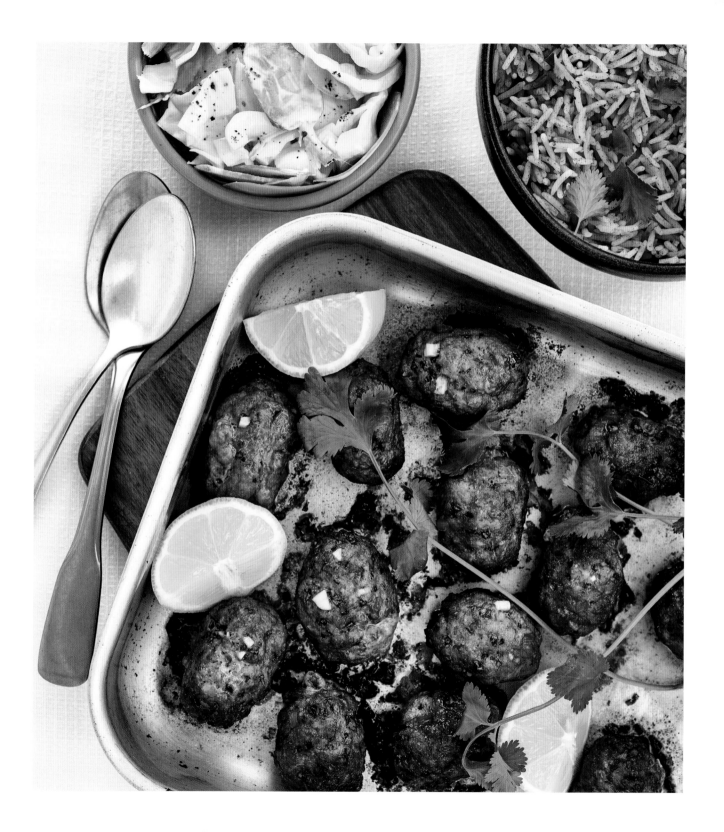

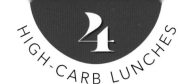

QUINOA, SWEET POTATO & BEETROOT SALAD WITH FETA

SERVES **2** ◆ PREP TIME **10 MINS** ◆ COOK TIME **30 MINS** ◆ DIFFICULTY **EASY** ◆ **GF** ◆ **V**

INGREDIENTS

1 large sweet potato
150g quinoa
1 avocado, peeled and chopped
2 carrots, peeled and grated or sliced into ribbons
6-8 cooked beetroots, quartered
2 tablespoons balsamic vinegar
80g feta cheese

JAMES SAYS: 'Don't worry about the sugar content in this recipe as it comes mostly from the vegetables.'

METHOD

1. Preheat your oven to 200°C. Wrap the sweet potato in foil and place whole into the oven. Bake the potato for 25-30 minutes or until cooked through. Remove the foil and allow to cool before touching. Carefully peel away the skin then cut the potato into 2cm dice and set aside.

2. Pour the quinoa into a sieve and wash under cold running water. Place in a saucepan, cover with water and add a pinch of salt. Bring to the boil then turn down to a simmer and cook for 12-15 minutes or until tender. Drain the quinoa and spread it out on a tray, moving it around with a fork to help it cool down. Once the quinoa has cooled, transfer it to a bowl.

3. Mix the avocado in with the quinoa. Then add in the carrots along with the sweet potato and the beetroots. Drizzle over the balsamic vinegar and give the salad a good toss. Divide between two plates, crumble the feta cheese over the top and serve.

PER SERVING

CARBS	ENERGY	FAT	SATURATES	PROTEIN	SUGAR	FIBRE	SALT
83g	691kcal	27g	9g	22g	27g	18g	1.5g

6 69014 44915 3

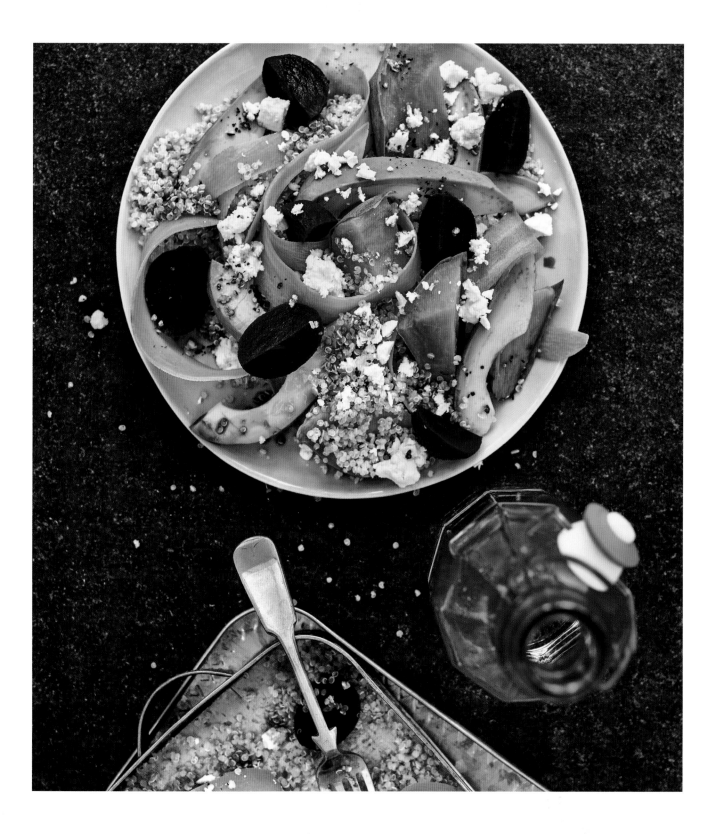

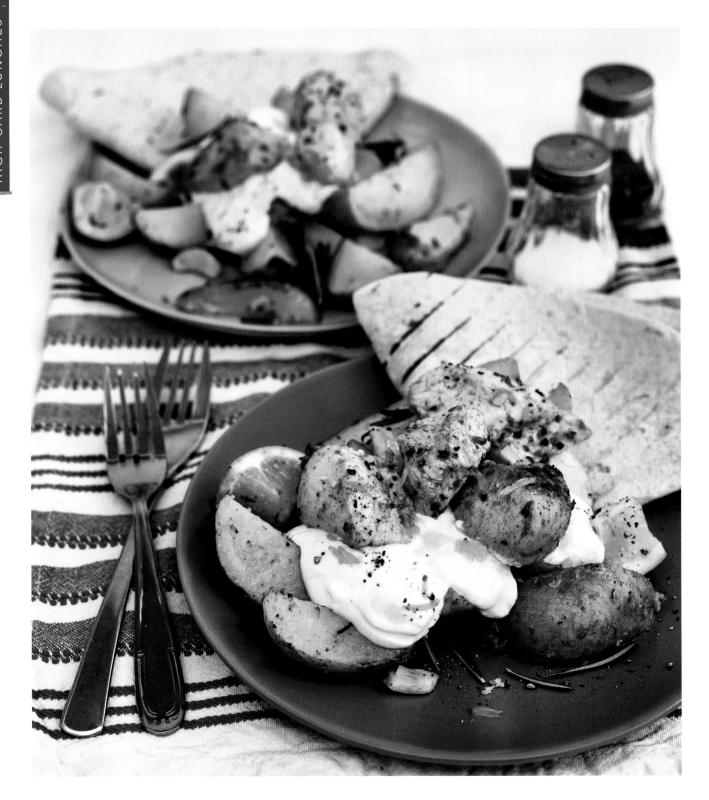

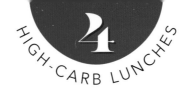
CHICKEN GYROS WITH LEMON POTATOES

SERVES **2** ◆ PREP TIME **5 MINS** ◆ COOK TIME **30 MINS** ◆ DIFFICULTY **EASY**

INGREDIENTS

CHICKEN
2 chicken breasts, skinless and boneless
2 garlic cloves, finely chopped
Zest and juice of 1 lemon
1 tablespoon olive oil
½ teaspoon ground cumin
½ teaspoon ground coriander
1 teaspoon dried oregano
½ teaspoon paprika

LEMON POTATOES
2 medium potatoes
3 garlic cloves, crushed
1 sprig rosemary
1 tablespoon olive oil
1 lemon
1 tablespoon fine polenta

2 flatbreads
2 tablespoons Greek yoghurt

METHOD

1. Preheat your oven to 200°C.

2. Chop each chicken breast into 4 pieces and place in a mixing bowl. Add the garlic, lemon zest and juice along with the olive oil, cumin, coriander, oregano, paprika and salt and pepper. Give this a good mix and place into the fridge for at least 30 minutes to marinate. Now place the chicken on a roasting tray and roast in the oven for 15 minutes or until cooked through.

3. Cut the potatoes into wedges and place on a roasting tray, along with the garlic and the rosemary. Drizzle over the olive oil and season with salt and pepper. Zest the lemon over the potatoes then roughly chop the lemon and add to the roasting tray. Sprinkle the polenta over the wedges and give the whole tray a good mix. Pop into the oven and bake for 25-30 minutes or until cooked through and crunchy on the outside.

4. Serve the potatoes with the chicken and the flatbreads, topped with a spoonful of Greek yoghurt.

PER SERVING

CARBS	ENERGY	FAT	SATURATES	PROTEIN	SUGAR	FIBRE	SALT
68g	635 kcal	18g	3.5g	46g	4g	6g	0.9g

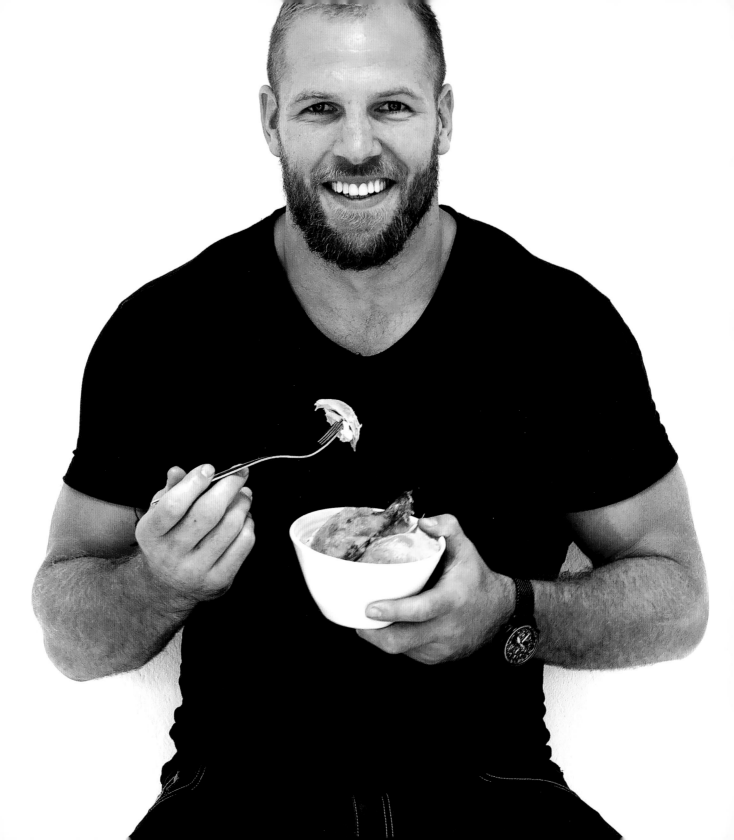

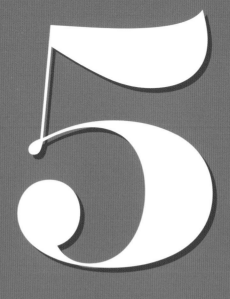

5

LOW-CARB DINNERS

From a hearty Sunday roast
to a clever twist on lasagne,
these dishes are so delicious
you'll hardly notice that you're
actually eating fewer
carbs.

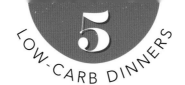

FILLET STEAK WITH PARSNIP MASH & WATERCRESS

SERVES **2** ◆ PREP TIME **5 MINS** ◆ COOK TIME **25 MINS** ◆ DIFFICULTY **EASY** ◆ **GF**

INGREDIENTS

2 x 175g-225g fillet steaks
1 tablespoon olive oil
2 bunches watercress

PARSNIP MASH

4 large parsnips, peeled and chopped
350ml semi-skimmed milk
1 teaspoon ground cumin
1 pinch ground nutmeg
2 knobs of butter

JAMES SAYS: 'For an even lower-carb option use mashed cauliflower instead.'

METHOD

1. First make the parsnip mash. Place the parsnips in a medium saucepan and pour over the milk. Add the cumin, nutmeg and butter. Heat the pan over a medium heat and cook for 15 minutes or until the parsnips are very soft all the way through. Scoop out the parsnips, place them in a food processor and blend, slowly adding some of the milk bit by bit until you have the consistency of mashed potato. Adjust the seasoning, transfer the mash to a saucepan and keep warm.

2. Season the steaks with salt and pepper and rub them with the olive oil. Heat a frying pan over a medium-high heat and add the steaks. Cook for 2-3 minutes on each side and then colour the sides of the steaks. Once the steaks are cooked allow them to rest for at least 5 minutes.

3. To serve, spoon the parsnip mash onto the centre of two serving plates. Slice the steak and serve on top of the mash. Place a bunch of watercress next to each steak and serve.

PER SERVING

CARBS	ENERGY	FAT	SATURATES	PROTEIN	SUGAR	FIBRE	SALT
44g	662kcal	27g	11g	50g	25g	15.5g	0.7g

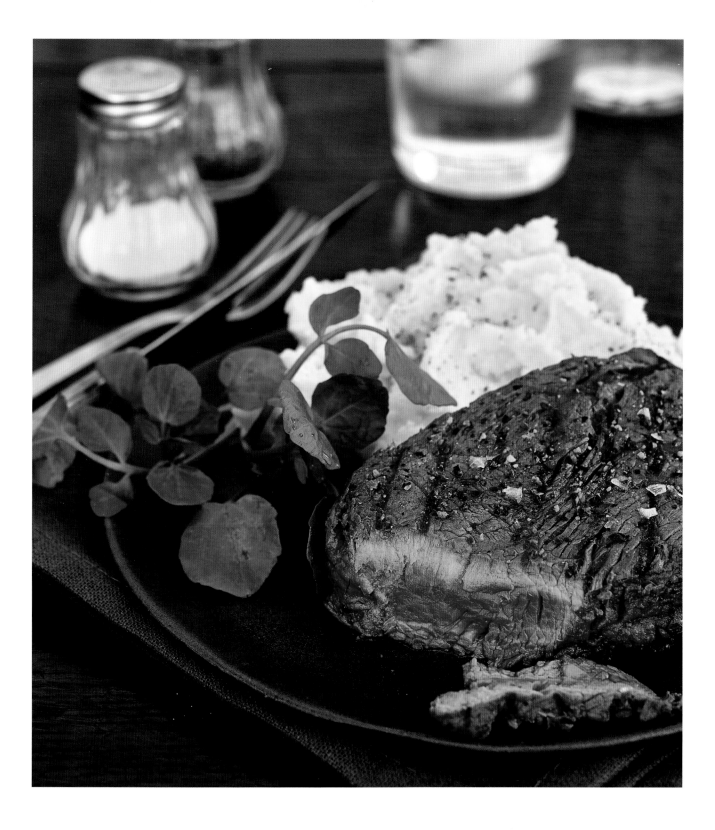

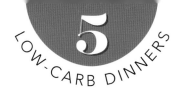

JAMES'S LOW-CARB SUNDAY ROAST

SERVES **4** ◆ PREP TIME **15 MINS** ◆ COOK TIME **1 HR 10 MINS** ◆ DIFFICULTY **MODERATE**

INGREDIENTS

1 whole chicken, 1.5kg-2kg
1 lemon, halved
1 small bunch thyme
1 whole garlic bulb
8 medium parsnips, peeled and cut into batons
1 tablespoon olive oil
1 tablespoon polenta
1 knob of butter
4 rashers streaky bacon, sliced
½ savoy cabbage, finely shredded
1 pinch nutmeg
½ cauliflower, cut into wedges

GRAVY
1 glass good quality red wine
1 sprig thyme
300ml chicken stock

METHOD

1. Preheat your oven to 200°C.

2. Season the chicken both inside and out with salt and pepper. Stuff the lemon and thyme into the chicken. Reserve 2 of the garlic cloves and stuff the rest into the chicken. Place the chicken on a roasting tray, and cover loosely with tin foil. Roast in the oven for 50 minutes. Now turn the oven down to 170°C, remove the foil and cook for another 30 minutes. Check the chicken is cooked by piercing the thigh with a sharp knife. The juices should run clear. Once cooked, allow the chicken to rest for 15-20 minutes.

3. Meanwhile, place the parsnips in a saucepan and cover with water. Bring to the boil and cook for 5 minutes. Drain the parsnips and place on a roasting tray. Season with salt and pepper and drizzle over the olive oil. Give them a dusting of polenta and roast in the oven for 20 minutes until crispy and golden brown.

4. Melt the butter in a saucepan over a high heat and add 1 whole garlic clove. Add the bacon to the pan and cook until golden brown. Now add the cabbage, season with salt and pepper then cook for 5 minutes or until the cabbage is softened. Season with nutmeg and set aside. Half-fill a saucepan with water and bring to the boil. Add the cauliflower wedges and cook for 2-3 minutes. Drain and set aside.

5. To make the gravy, pour the red wine into a saucepan along with the thyme and 1 garlic clove and bring to the boil. When the wine has reduced by half pour in the chicken stock. Bring back to the boil, reduce by half again and set aside.

6. Carve the chicken, serve with the vegetables, with the gravy alongside.

PER SERVING

CARBS	ENERGY	FAT	SATURATES	PROTEIN	SUGAR	FIBRE	SALT
35g	685 kcal	32g	7g	68g	16g	14g	1.4g

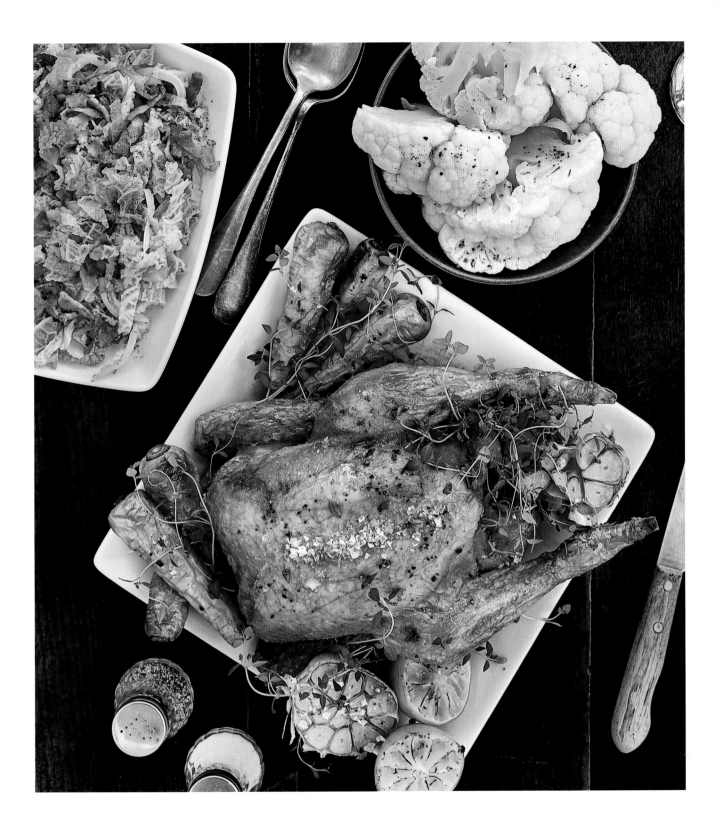

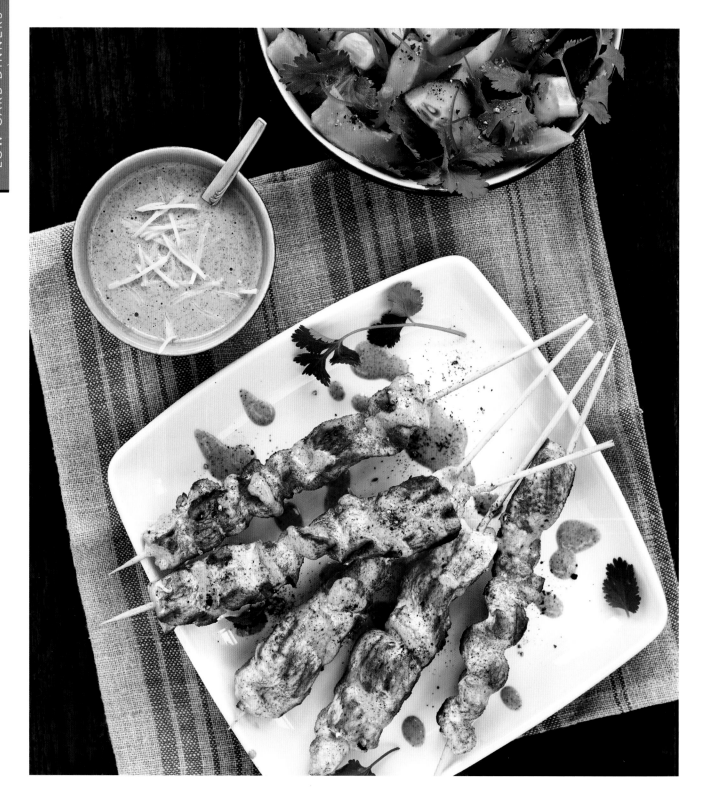

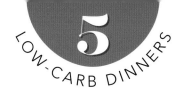

SATAY CHICKEN WITH PAPAYA & CHILLI SALAD

SERVES **2** ◆ PREP TIME **10 MINS** ◆ COOK TIME **20 MINS** ◆ DIFFICULTY **EASY** ◆ **GF** ◆ **DF**

INGREDIENTS

2 chicken breasts, skinless and
boneless
1 tablespoon curry powder
1 tablespoon olive oil

SATAY SAUCE
Juice of 1 lime
4 tablespoons Meridian Peanut
Butter
½cm piece of ginger
1 red chilli
1 tablespoon curry powder
1 garlic clove, peeled
1 tablespoon tamari
1 teaspoon honey

PAPAYA SALAD
1 papaya, peeled and diced
1 cucumber, diced
½ red onion, finely chopped
½ red chilli, finely chopped
1 small bunch coriander
You will also need 4 kebab sticks

METHOD

1. Preheat your oven to 200°C.
2. Slice each chicken breast into 4 strips lengthways. Place them in a bowl and mix with the curry powder and olive oil. Chill in the fridge for at least 30 minutes. Now skewer the strips of chicken onto each kebab stick. Roast the chicken in the oven for 12-15 minutes or until cooked through. Allow to rest for 2 minutes.
3. Place all the ingredients for the satay sauce in a food processor along with 100ml water and blend until smooth. Set aside.
4. Place the papaya in a mixing bowl along with the cucumber, red onion and chilli. Roughly chop the coriander and mix everything together. Divide the salad between two plates and top with the chicken kebabs. Pour the satay sauce over the chicken and salad and serve.

PER SERVING

CARBS	ENERGY	FAT	SATURATES	PROTEIN	SUGAR	FIBRE	SALT
26g	540 kcal	24g	4g	49g	20g	13g	1.5g

6 69014 44919 1

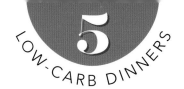

COURGETTE BEEF LASAGNE

SERVES **4** ◆ PREP TIME **10 MINS** ◆ COOK TIME **1 HR** ◆ DIFFICULTY **MODERATE**

INGREDIENTS

3 tablespoons olive oil
1 onion, finely chopped
2 garlic cloves, finely chopped
500g lean beef mince
1 pinch ground cumin
1 pinch ground cinnamon
400g tin chopped tomatoes
2 tablespoons tomato purée
150ml water
6 courgettes
4 tablespoons grated Parmesan

WHITE SAUCE
50g butter
50g plain flour
300ml semi-skimmed milk
400ml water
1 pinch nutmeg

JAMES SAYS: 'I love lasagne so it's great to have this low-carb alternative.'

METHOD

1. Preheat your oven to 200°C.

2. Heat 1 tablespoon of the olive oil in a large saucepan over a high heat. Add the onion and garlic to the pan, and cook for 1 minute without colouring. Add the beef to the pan and cook for 5 minutes or until browned all over. Add the cumin and cinnamon and stir well. Pour over the chopped tomatoes, tomato purée and water, and turn the heat down to a gentle simmer. Continue cooking for 15-20 minutes. Remove from the heat and allow to cool slightly. Check the seasoning and add salt and pepper if needed.

3. For the white sauce, melt the butter in a large saucepan over a medium heat. Next whisk in the flour. Add the milk and water and whisk until combined and smooth. Simmer the sauce for 10 minutes, whisking continuously. Season with salt and pepper and add a pinch of nutmeg.

4. Slice the courgettes lengthways into ribbons, roughly ⅓cm thick. Lay the courgette ribbons out on a baking tray and drizzle with the remaining olive oil, season with salt and pepper and pop into the oven for 5 minutes or until slightly softened.

5. To arrange the lasagne, spoon some of the beef into the bottom of a baking dish, top with a layer of courgette ribbons and then another ladleful of beef, then top again with courgette ribbons. Now pour over the white sauce and sprinkle over the Parmesan cheese. Pop into the oven and cook for 20 minutes or until golden brown and crispy on top.

PER SERVING

CARBS	ENERGY	FAT	SATURATES	PROTEIN	SUGAR	FIBRE	SALT
26g	551kcal	29g	13g	44g	15g	6g	0.8g

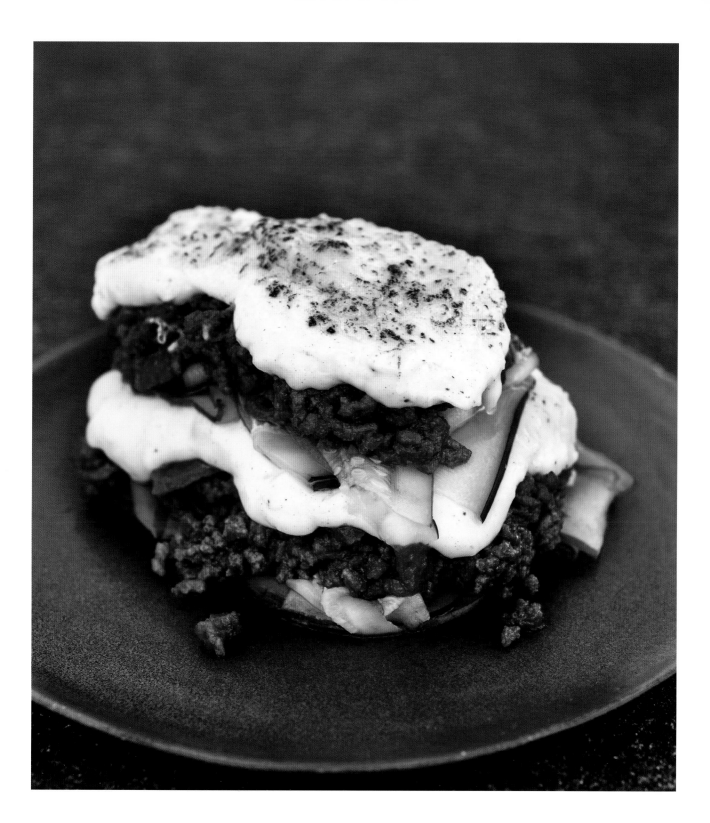

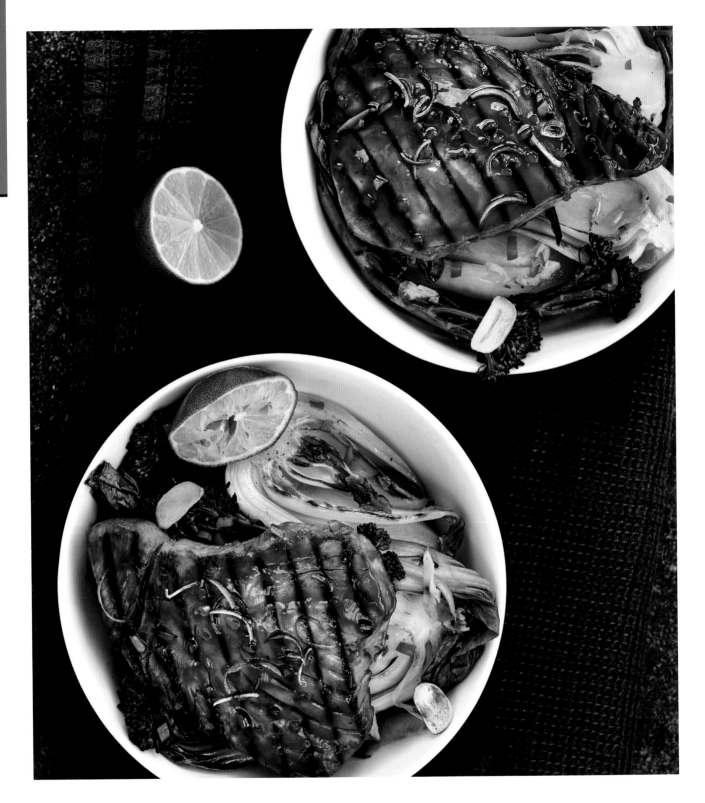

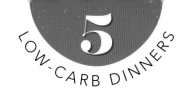

TERIYAKI-GLAZED TUNA WITH STIR-FRIED PAK CHOI

SERVES **2** ◆ PREP TIME **10 MINS** ◆ COOK TIME **15 MINS** ◆ DIFFICULTY **EASY** ◆ **DF**

INGREDIENTS

4-5 tablespoons teriyaki sauce
½ red chilli, finely chopped
1 garlic clove, finely chopped
Zest and juice of 1 lime
2 tuna steaks, about 200g each
1 tablespoon sesame oil
2 small pak choi, sliced into quarters lengthways
4-5 tender stem broccoli florets, cut into thirds
½cm piece ginger, finely chopped
1 red chilli, finely chopped
1 garlic clove, finely chopped

OMAR SAYS: 'This also works well with salmon fillets or chicken breasts.'

METHOD

1. Preheat your oven to 200°C.

2. Pour the teriyaki sauce into a small bowl and stir in the chilli and garlic. Mix in the lime zest and juice. Place the tuna steaks on a small oven tray and spoon over half of the sauce. Pop the tuna into the oven for 8 minutes or until the fish is cooked through.

3. Heat a wok over a high heat. Carefully add the sesame oil. Now add the pak choi and broccoli and stir-fry for 2-3 minutes, ensuring you are moving the pan constantly. Now toss in the ginger, chilli and garlic and cook for a further 1 minute. Once cooked divide between 2 serving bowls.

4. Top the pak choi with the tuna steaks and spoon over the remaining teriyaki sauce.

PER SERVING

CARBS	ENERGY	FAT	SATURATES	PROTEIN	SUGAR	FIBRE	SALT
17.5g	360 kcal	7g	1.5g	54g	16.5g	3.5g	2.6g

6 69014 44921 4

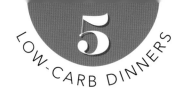

BEAN FALAFEL WITH KALETTE & APPLE SALAD

SERVES **2** ◆ PREP TIME **15 MINS** ◆ COOK TIME **15 MINS** ◆ DIFFICULTY **EASY** ◆ **V**

INGREDIENTS

FALAFEL
200g cooked kidney beans
200g cooked butter beans
2 garlic cloves
1 tablespoon Meridian Almond Butter
1 teaspoon cayenne pepper
1 teaspoon Cajun seasoning

SALAD
1 knob of butter
150g Kalettes, halved
1 green apple, cored and sliced
10 radishes

DRESSING
4 tablespoons Greek yoghurt
2 tablespoons white wine vinegar
½ red chilli
½ bunch flat-leaf parsley

OMAR SAYS: 'You can use curly kale or brussels sprouts instead of Kalettes.'

METHOD

1. Preheat your oven to 200°C.

2. Place the ingredients for the falafel in a food processor and pulse until you have a paste that comes together. Now roll the paste into 8 small balls and place on a lined roasting tray. Pop into the oven and bake for 12 minutes. Allow to cool for 5 minutes.

3. Melt the butter in a frying pan over a high heat. Add the Kalettes and cook for 2 minutes. Transfer to a mixing bowl and add the apple and radishes. Divide the salad between 2 serving plates.

4. Place the ingredients for the dressing in a food processor and blend until smooth.

5. To serve, place the falafel on the salad and pour over the yoghurt dressing.

PER SERVING

CARBS	ENERGY	FAT	SATURATES	PROTEIN	SUGAR	FIBRE	SALT
44.5g	437 kcal	14g	5.5g	22.5g	12g	21g	0.8g

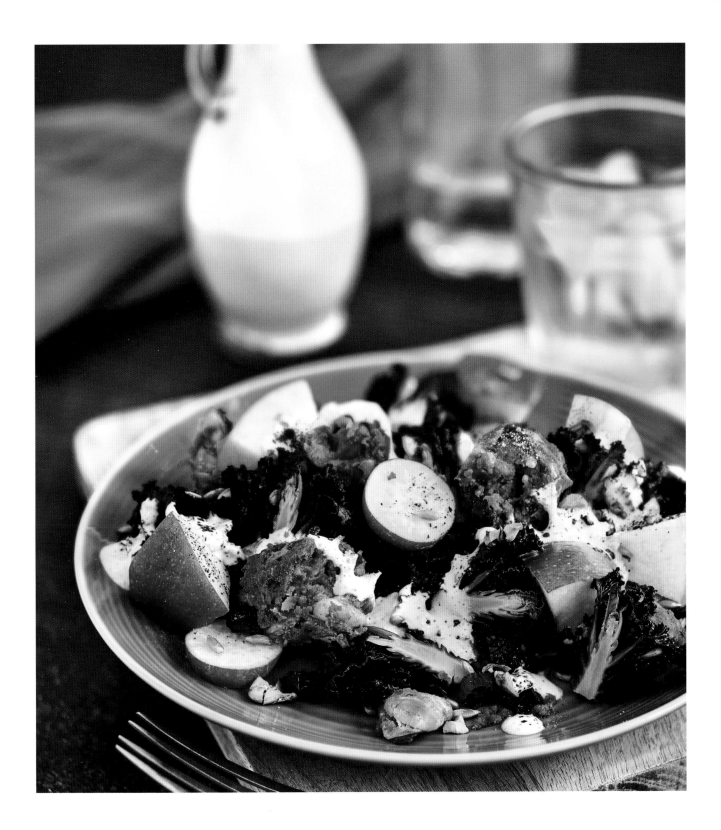

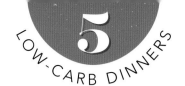

CURRIED PORK CHOP WITH INDIAN CUCUMBER SALAD

SERVES **2** ◆ PREP TIME **15 MINS** ◆ COOK TIME **15 MINS** ◆ DIFFICULTY **EASY** ◆ **GF**

INGREDIENTS

2 large pork chops
1 tablespoon tikka masala seasoning
1 tablespoon olive oil

CUCUMBER SALAD

½ cucumber, diced
1 beef tomato, diced
3 spring onions, finely sliced
1 red onion, finely sliced
1 small bunch coriander, finely chopped
1 pinch ground cumin
1 pinch ground cinnamon
2 tablespoons Greek yoghurt

METHOD

1. Preheat your oven to 180°C.

2. Place the chops in a large bowl and add the tikka masala seasoning and olive oil. Give it a good mix before popping it into the fridge for at least 30 minutes. Once the pork has marinated place on an oven tray and bake in the oven for 10-12 minutes or until cooked through.

3. Place the cucumber, tomato, spring onions and red onion in a bowl. Add the finely chopped coriander along with the cumin and cinnamon and mix well. Season with salt and pepper then divide between 2 serving plates.

4. Once the pork is cooked allow to rest for 5 minutes before serving alongside the cucumber salad. Top with a dollop of Greek yoghurt.

PER SERVING

CARBS	ENERGY	FAT	SATURATES	PROTEIN	SUGAR	FIBRE	SALT
12g	365 kcal	15.5g	4.5g	42g	9g	5.5g	0.4g

6 69014 44923 8

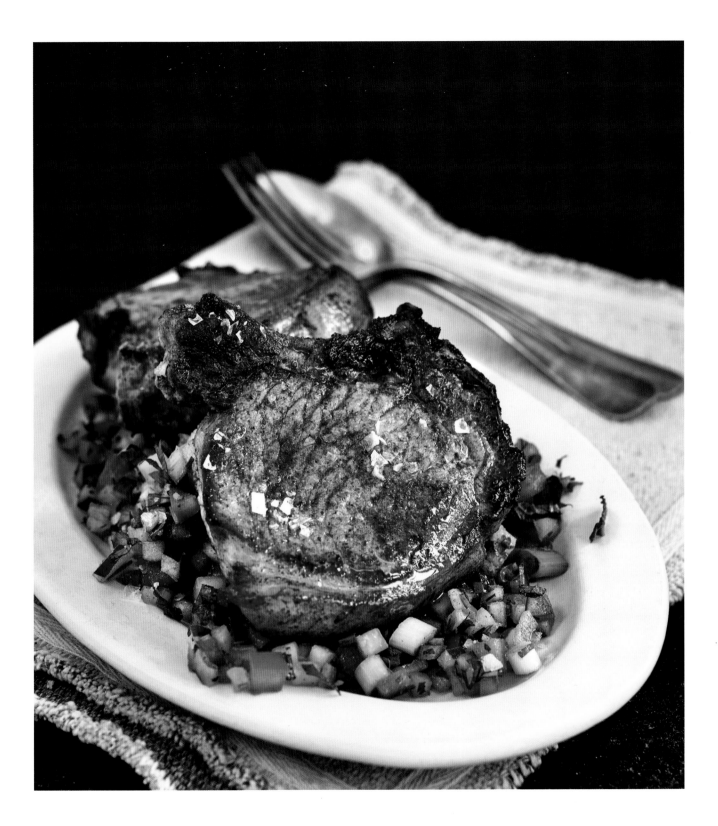

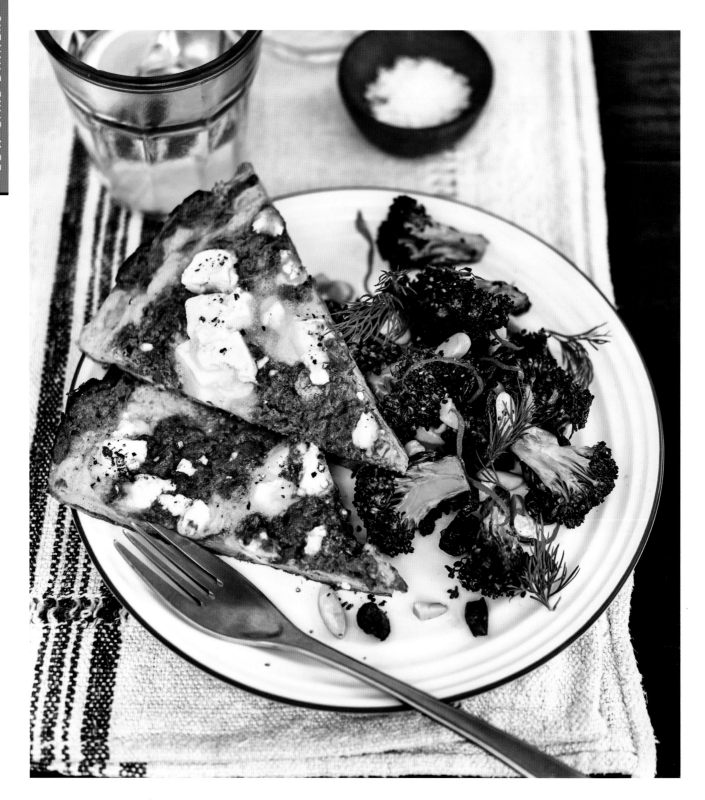

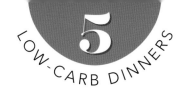
PESTO & FETA FRITTATA WITH ROASTED BROCCOLI SALAD

SERVES **2** ◆ PREP TIME **15 MINS** ◆ COOK TIME **25 MINS** ◆ DIFFICULTY **EASY** ◆ **GF**

INGREDIENTS

6 large eggs
1 knob of butter
100g feta cheese
2 tablespoons basil pesto

BROCCOLI SALAD

1 medium head of broccoli, cut into florets
1 tablespoon olive oil
½ red chilli, finely chopped
½ small bunch dill, finely chopped
2 tablespoons dried cranberries
1 tablespoon whole almonds

JAMES SAYS: 'The flavour combination of feta and basil makes this taste amazing.'

METHOD

1. Preheat your oven to 180°C.

2. First make the broccoli salad. Place the broccoli florets on a roasting tray. Season with salt and pepper and drizzle over the olive oil. Roast in the oven for 10 minutes or until the broccoli is browning and cooked through, but with a slight crunch. Remove from the oven and allow to cool. Mix the chilli and the dill together with the broccoli. Sprinkle over the cranberries and almonds, then divide between two serving plates.

3. Crack the eggs into a bowl and season with salt and pepper. Whisk the eggs together. Melt the butter in a frying pan over a medium heat and add the whisked eggs. Crumble the feta into the eggs and ensure it is evenly dispersed. With a teaspoon dot the pesto around the frittata and then pop into the oven. Bake for 10-12 minutes or until cooked through. Once the frittata is cooked remove from the oven and allow to cool slightly before slicing into wedges and serving alongside the salad.

PER SERVING

CARBS	ENERGY	FAT	SATURATES	PROTEIN	SUGAR	FIBRE	SALT
16.5g	650 kcal	46g	14.5g	41g	14g	5g	2.4g

6 69014 44924 5

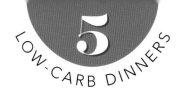

LAMB CHOPS WITH ROASTED VEGETABLES & SALSA VERDE

SERVES **2** ◆ PREP TIME **15 MINS** ◆ COOK TIME **20 MINS** ◆ DIFFICULTY **EASY** ◆ **GF** ◆ **DF**

INGREDIENTS

4 lamb chops
Zest and juice of 1 lemon
5 garlic cloves
1 head of fennel, sliced into 6 wedges
1 red pepper, chopped
1 red onion, chopped into 6 wedges
2 courgettes, chopped
1 tablespoon olive oil

SALSA VERDE

1 bunch flat-leaf parsley
10 mint leaves
2 garlic cloves
2 tablespoons capers
3 tablespoons olive oil
1 teaspoon Dijon mustard
1 teaspoon white wine vinegar

METHOD

1. Preheat your oven to 200°C.

2. Place the lamb chops in a bowl and sprinkle the lemon zest and juice over them. Finely chop 4 of the garlic cloves, mix them with the lamb chops and leave to marinate for 10 minutes.

3. Place the fennel, red pepper, onion and courgettes on a roasting tray. Finely chop the remaining garlic clove and mix together with the vegetables. Drizzle over the olive oil, season with salt and pepper and roast in the oven for 12-15 minutes.

4. Place all the ingredients for the salsa verde in a food processor and blend until everything is combined. You still want the salsa slightly chunky.

5. Place the lamb chops on a roasting tray and roast in the oven for 10-12 minutes. Once the chops are cooked allow them to rest for 5 minutes before serving.

6. To serve, divide the roasted vegetables between 2 serving plates and top with the lamb chops. Spoon over the salsa verde.

PER SERVING

CARBS	ENERGY	FAT	SATURATES	PROTEIN	SUGAR	FIBRE	SALT
13g	677 kcal	43g	12g	55g	11g	8g	0.7g

6 69014 44925 2

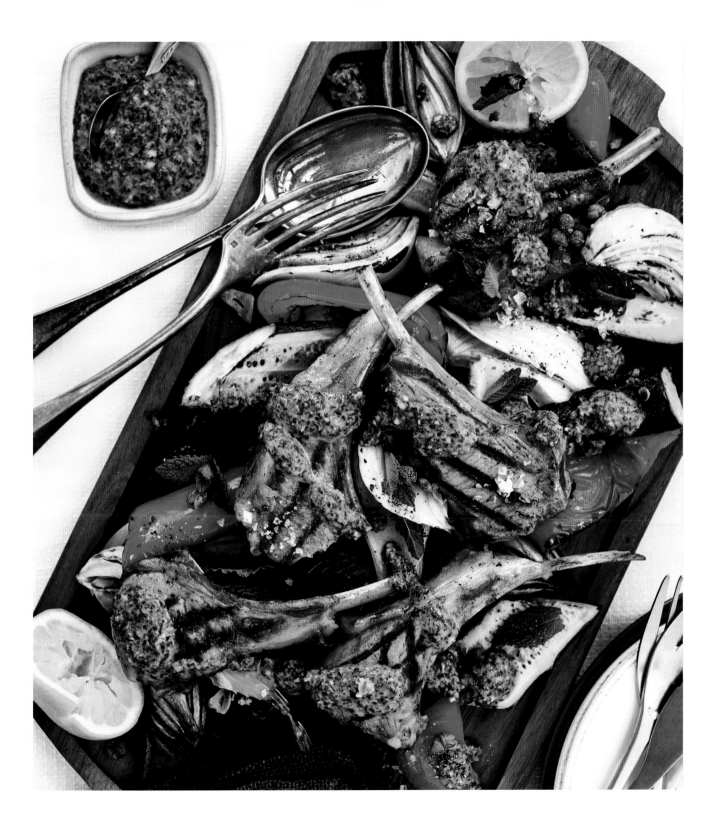

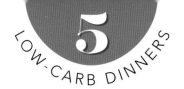

ROASTED DUCK WITH MOLASSES & AUBERGINE SALAD

SERVES **2** ◆ PREP TIME **5 MINS** ◆ COOK TIME **20 MINS** ◆ DIFFICULTY **MODERATE** ◆ **GF**

INGREDIENTS

2 duck breasts, skinless
4 sprigs thyme
2 tablespoons Meridian Molasses

AUBERGINE SALAD

1 large aubergine, cut into 2cm slices
1 tablespoon olive oil
1 pomegranate, cut in half and seeds removed
2 tablespoons Greek yoghurt
1 small bunch dill, roughly chopped
Zest of 1 lemon
50g feta cheese
1 tablespoon Meridian Date Syrup

METHOD

1. Preheat your oven to 180°C.

2. First make the aubergine salad. Heat a large frying pan over a high heat. Place the aubergine slices in a large bowl. Drizzle over the olive oil and season with salt and pepper. Carefully add the aubergine to the hot pan and cook for 2-3 minutes on each side or until browned. Place in a Tupperware container with the lid on for at least 5 minutes.

3. Lay the aubergine slices on a serving plate and scatter the pomegranate seeds over the top. Spoon over the yoghurt then add the dill and lemon zest. Crumble the feta cheese over the top and set the salad aside.

4. Heat another frying pan over a medium heat. Season the duck breasts with salt and pepper and the sprigs of thyme. Add the duck to the pan and cook for 5-6 minutes until golden brown. Pour the fat from the pan into a jar (to use another time), turn the duck breasts over and cook for 1 minute.

5. Transfer the duck to a roasting tray, pour over the molasses and roast in the oven for 6-7 minutes. Once the duck is cooked allow it to rest for 5 minutes before slicing and dividing between 2 serving plates. Spoon over the molasses from the bottom of the roasting tray and serve with the aubergine salad. Drizzle over the date syrup.

PER SERVING

CARBS	ENERGY	FAT	SATURATES	PROTEIN	SUGAR	FIBRE	SALT
20g	480 kcal	24g	9g	41g	23g	7g	1.2g

6 69014 44926 9

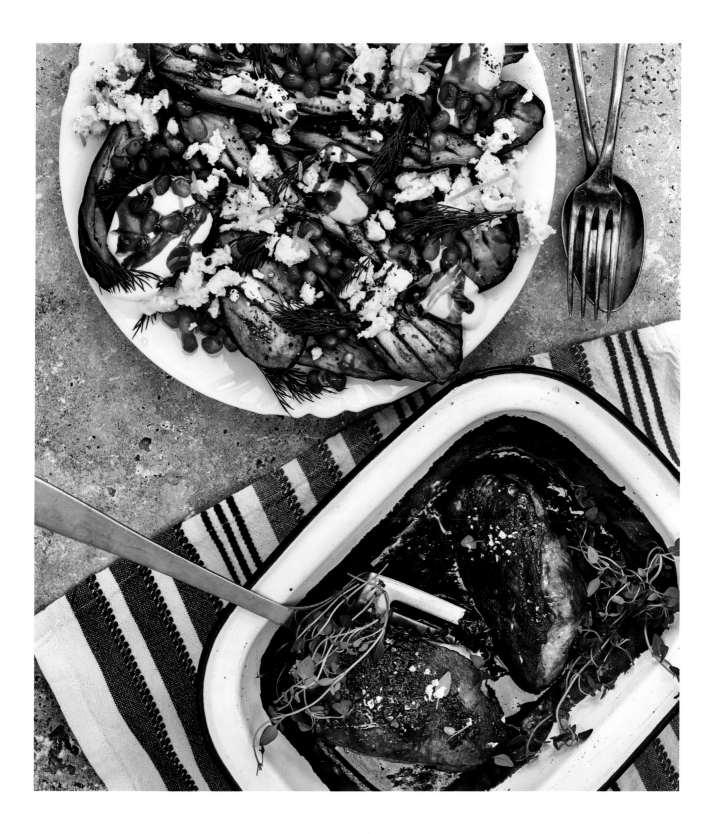

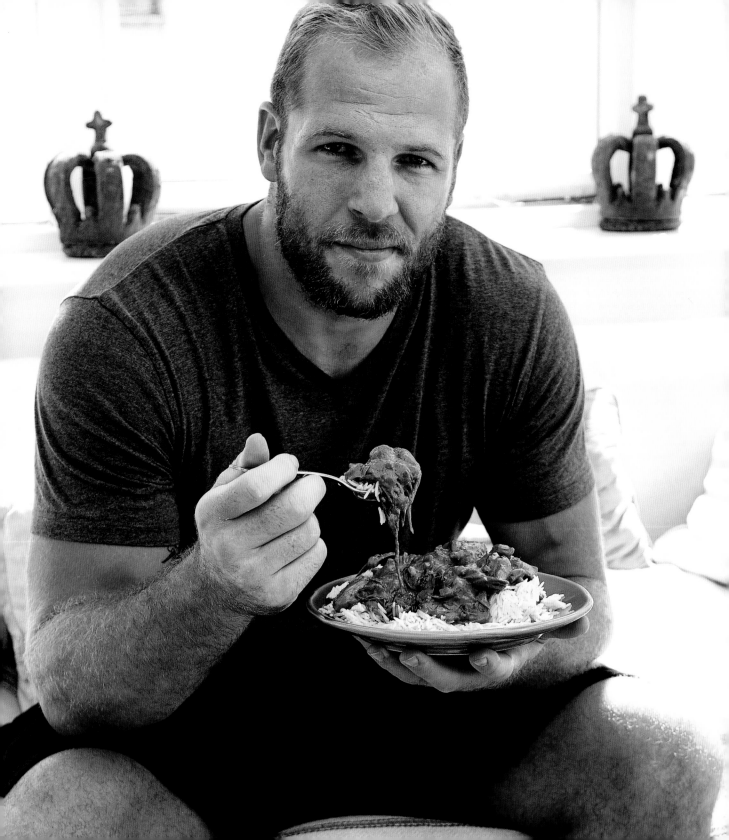

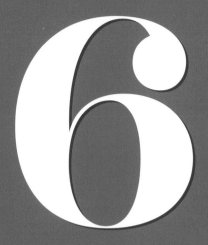

6

HIGH-CARB
DINNERS

These are some of my favourite
meals to cook after a tough day's
training or match. Remember,
you can only build muscle by
eating plenty of healthy carbs
and protein.

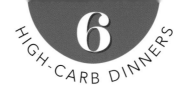

JAMES'S FISH & CHIPS

SERVES **2** ◆ PREP TIME **20 MINS** ◆ COOK TIME **30 MINS** ◆ DIFFICULTY **EASY** ◆ **DF**

INGREDIENTS

2 large Maris Piper potatoes
2 tablespoons olive oil
2 tablespoons fine polenta
2 eggs
8 heaped tablespoons panko breadcrumbs
2 heaped tablespoons plain flour
2 salmon fillets, about 150g each
1 lemon, cut into wedges

JAMES SAYS: 'This home-made version of fish and chips has much less saturated fat and tastes better too.'

METHOD

1. Preheat your oven to 200°C.

2. Give the potatoes a good wash but don't peel them. Chop into thick chips and place in a saucepan. Cover with cold water, bring to the boil over a high heat and cook for 5 minutes. Drain the potatoes in a colander and leave for 5 minutes to dry. Place the potatoes on a roasting tray and drizzle over the olive oil and season with salt and pepper. Now sprinkle over the polenta and give them a good mix. Bake the potatoes in the oven for 20-25 minutes or until crunchy and cooked through.

3. Meanwhile, whisk the eggs in a bowl and season with salt and pepper. Place the breadcrumbs in a bowl and pour the flour into another bowl. Dip the salmon into the flour, shake off any excess then place the salmon into the egg before dipping into the breadcrumbs. Ensure the fish are completely covered in breadcrumbs. Place the fish on a baking tray and pop into the oven for 10-12 minutes or until the salmon is cooked through.

4. Divide the chips and salmon between 2 plates. Serve with lemon wedges to squeeze over the fish.

PER SERVING

CARBS	ENERGY	FAT	SATURATES	PROTEIN	SUGAR	FIBRE	SALT
98g	947 kcal	39g	7g	48g	4g	7g	0.85g

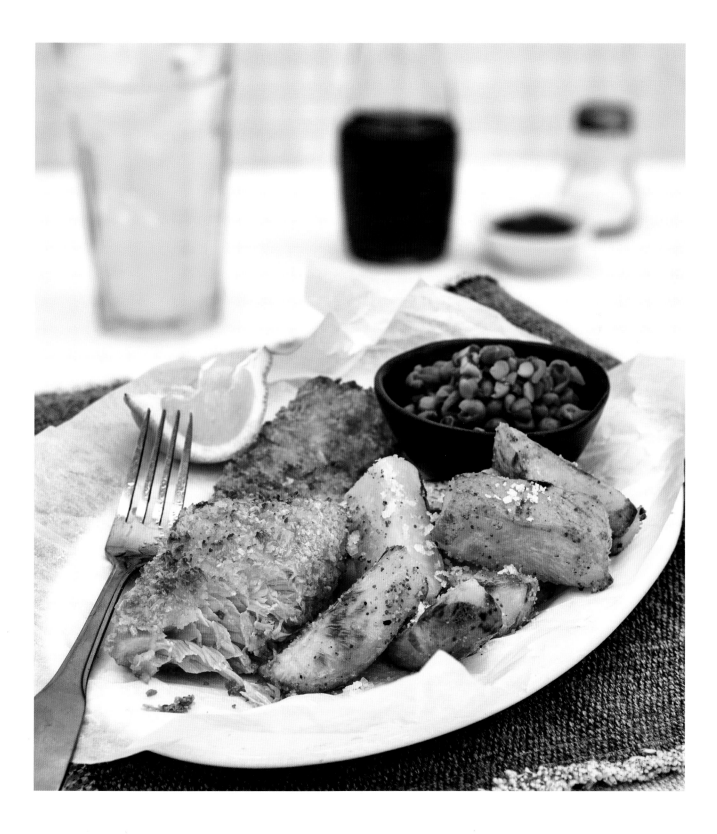

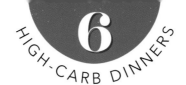

SEA BASS WITH GINGER & TAMARI, BOILED RICE & EDAMAME BEANS

SERVES **2** ◆ PREP TIME **10 MINS** ◆ COOK TIME **35 MINS** ◆ DIFFICULTY **EASY** ◆ **DF**

INGREDIENTS

180g brown rice
80g edamame beans
½ small bunch coriander, finely chopped
2 whole sea bass
2 garlic cloves, finely chopped
1cm piece of ginger, finely chopped
1 red chilli, finely chopped
3 tablespoons tamari or soy sauce
4 spring onions, finely chopped

OMAR SAYS: 'You'll know the whole fish is cooked through when the backbone can be removed easily, pulling it away by the tail first.'

METHOD

1. Preheat your grill to high.

2. Place the rice in a saucepan and cover with water. Bring to the boil and cook for 10 minutes or according to the pack instructions. Drain away any excess water and put the rice back into the saucepan and set aside. Now bring a small saucepan of water to the boil and carefully add the edamame beans. Boil the beans for 5 minutes before draining and mixing together with the rice. Stir in the finely chopped coriander.

3. Place the sea bass on a roasting tray skin-side up. Sprinkle the garlic, ginger and chilli over the fish. Spoon over the tamari and place under the hot grill. Cook for 15 minutes. Baste the fish with the sauce in the roasting tray.

4. Divide the rice between 2 plates and top with the fish. Spoon over any excess sauce. Scatter the spring onions over the fish and serve.

PER SERVING

CARBS	ENERGY	FAT	SATURATES	PROTEIN	SUGAR	FIBRE	SALT
75g	830 kcal	29g	6g	63g	6g	5g	3.5g

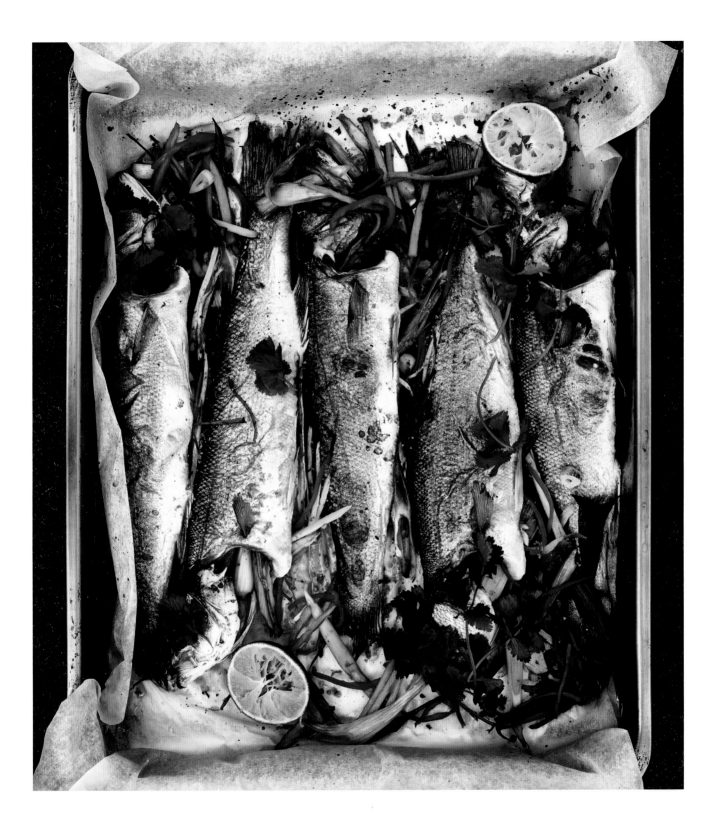

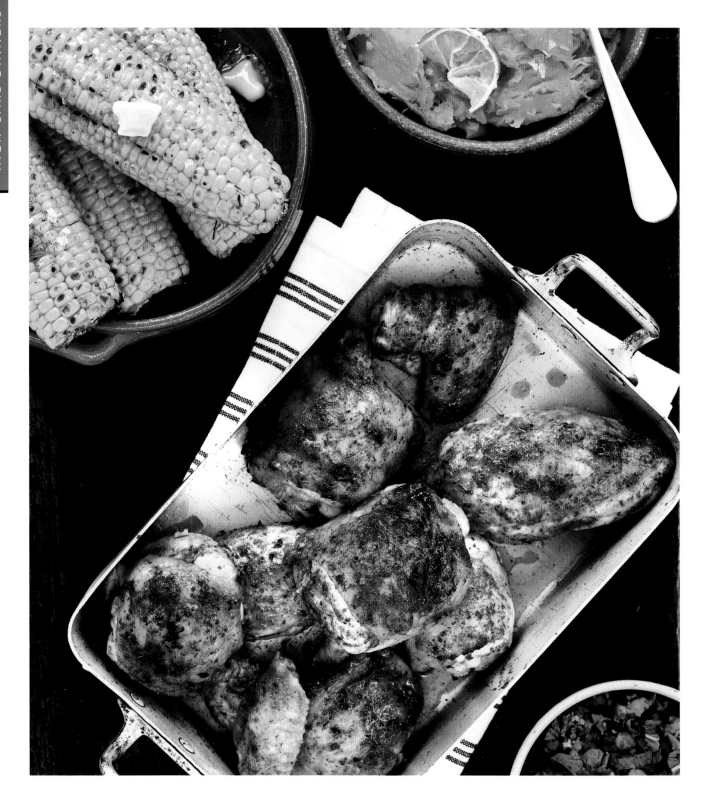

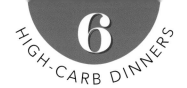
PERI-PERI CHICKEN FEAST

SERVES **2** ◆ PREP TIME **15 MINS** ◆ COOK TIME **1 HR** ◆ DIFFICULTY **EASY** ◆ **GF** ◆ **DF**

INGREDIENTS

2 medium sweet potatoes
Juice of 1 lime
2 chicken breasts plus 2 chicken thighs, skinless and boneless
1 tablespoon olive oil
2 tablespoons peri-peri seasoning
2 whole corn cobs

MACHO PEAS
350g peas
½ red chilli, finely chopped
10 mint leaves, finely chopped

JAMES SAYS: 'This is great with some Greek yoghurt mixed with Cajun spices.'

METHOD

1. Preheat your oven to 180°C.

2. Place the potatoes on a roasting tray and bake for 25-30 minutes. Once the potatoes are cooked remove from the oven and allow to rest for 10 minutes. Now slice the potatoes down the centre and peel away the skin. Place in a mixing bowl and mash with a fork. Season with salt and pepper and add the lime juice. Set aside.

3. Place the chicken pieces on a roasting tray and drizzle over the olive oil. Sprinkle over the peri-peri seasoning and massage into the meat. Place the chicken in the oven and roast for 25 minutes or until cooked through.

4. Meanwhile, season the corn cobs with salt and pepper and place on a roasting tray. Pop into the oven and bake for 15 minutes.

5. Half-fill a medium-sized saucepan with water and bring to the boil over a high heat. Carefully add the peas and cook for 2 minutes. Drain the peas and transfer to a bowl. Mix in the chilli and mint. Season with salt and pepper and gently crush with a potato masher.

6. To serve, divide the sweet potato mash, peas and corn between 2 plates. Dish up the chicken alongside the veg.

PER SERVING

CARBS	ENERGY	FAT	SATURATES	PROTEIN	SUGAR	FIBRE	SALT
68g	719 kcal	15g	3g	70g	17g	17g	0.8g

6 69014 44929 0

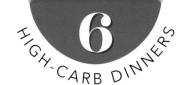

JAMES'S FISH PIE

SERVES **4** ◆ PREP TIME **15 MINS** ◆ COOK TIME **1 HR** ◆ DIFFICULTY **MODERATE**

INGREDIENTS

3 medium potatoes, peeled and cut
into ½cm slices
1 salmon fillet, about 150g
1 cod fillet, 150g-200g
8-10 king prawns, shells removed
2 large eggs
1 knob of butter
200g fresh spinach
100g peas

WHITE SAUCE
50g butter
50g plain flour
300ml semi-skimmed milk
400ml water
1 pinch nutmeg
You will also need a 22-25cm
pie dish

METHOD

1. Preheat your oven to 180°C.

2. Place the potato slices in a medium saucepan and cover with cold water. Bring to the boil and cook for 5 minutes. Drain and set aside.

3. Chop the salmon and cod into equal-sized pieces and place in a bowl along with the prawns. Season with salt and pepper.

4. Fill a small saucepan with water and bring to the boil over a high heat. Carefully place the eggs in the water. Once the water has begun to boil again start timing for 3 minutes. Drain the eggs and run under cold water. Peel away the shell and set the eggs aside.

5. Melt the butter in a large saucepan over a medium heat, add the spinach and season with salt and pepper. Cook the spinach for 1 minute or until wilted. Remove from the pan and allow to drain on kitchen paper.

6. For the white sauce, melt the butter in a large saucepan over a high heat. Add the flour and whisk together. Pour in the milk and water and whisk until smooth. Simmer the sauce for 10 minutes and season with salt and pepper and a pinch of nutmeg. Pour the sauce into a large mixing bowl and add the fish and prawns, the spinach and the peas. Slice the eggs and add them too.

7. Pour the mix into a pie dish. Lay the potatoes over the top, overlapping like fish scales. Season with salt and pepper and pop into the oven for 35 minutes. Once the pie is cooked serve immediately.

PER SERVING

CARBS	ENERGY	FAT	SATURATES	PROTEIN	SUGAR	FIBRE	SALT
46g	530kcal	22.5g	10g	34g	5.2g	6g	0.8g

6 69014 44930 6

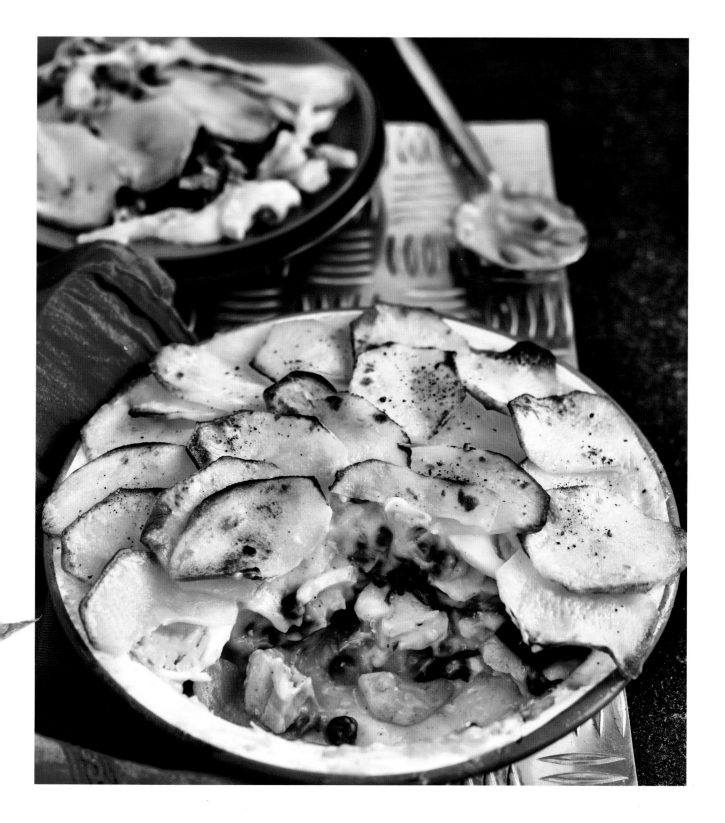

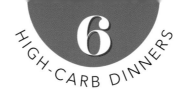

MASSAMAN BEEF CURRY

SERVES **2** ◆ PREP TIME **15 MINS** ◆ COOK TIME **1HR 40 MINS** ◆ DIFFICULTY **EASY** ◆ **GF** ◆ **DF**

INGREDIENTS

1 tablespoon coconut oil
350g diced beef (chuck steak)
200ml reduced-fat coconut milk
450ml cold water
2 Maris Piper potatoes, peeled
½ small bunch coriander, finely chopped
2 spring onions, finely chopped

CURRY PASTE

1 teaspoon ground cumin
½ teaspoon ground nutmeg
4 cloves
½ teaspoon ground cinnamon
1 tablespoon ground coriander
½ onion
1 tablespoon coconut oil
4 garlic cloves
½cm piece ginger
2-3 red chillies
1 tablespoon shrimp paste
Salt and pepper

METHOD

1. Place all the ingredients for the curry paste in a food processor and blend until you have a fine paste.

2. Heat the coconut oil in a large saucepan over a high heat. Carefully add the diced beef and season with salt and pepper. Cook the beef for 4-5 minutes ensuring it is browned all over. Now add the curry paste and continue to cook for 3-4 minutes, stirring continuously. Pour over the coconut milk and add the water. Bring the curry to the boil, before turning down to a gentle simmer. Cook the curry for 1 hour.

3. Cut each potato into 4 wedges and add them to the curry. Continue to cook the curry for 30 minutes or until the potatoes are cooked through and the beef is tender. Sprinkle the coriander and spring onions over the top of the curry and serve.

PER SERVING

CARBS	ENERGY	FAT	SATURATES	PROTEIN	SUGAR	FIBRE	SALT
42g	629 kcal	29g	20g	44g	6g	8g	1.6g

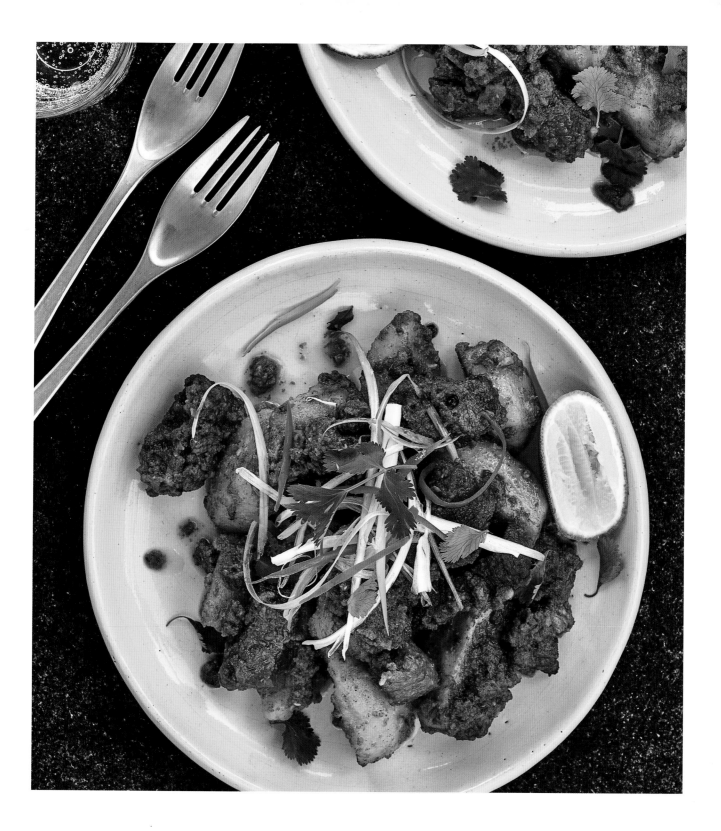

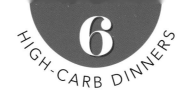
CURRIED TURKEY BURGER WITH SWEET POTATO WEDGES

SERVES **2** ◆ PREP TIME **15 MINS** ◆ COOK TIME **30 MINS** ◆ DIFFICULTY **EASY** ◆ **DF**

INGREDIENTS

360g turkey mince
1 tablespoon medium curry powder
2 garlic cloves, finely chopped
1 large sweet potato or 2 medium potatoes
1 pinch ground cumin
1 pinch ground cinnamon
2 tablespoons olive oil
2 ciabatta rolls
1 tablespoon mayonnaise
1 tomato, cut into 4 slices

OMAR SAYS: 'The burgers are cooked properly when there is no pink meat inside.'

METHOD

1. Preheat your oven to 200°C. Place the turkey mince in a large bowl and mix together with the curry powder. Stir in the garlic, season with salt and pepper, and mix thoroughly. Form into 2 burgers and place in the fridge for 30 minutes.

2. Cut the potato into wedges and lay out on a roasting tray. Season with salt and pepper and sprinkle over the cumin and cinnamon. Drizzle over half the olive oil and give the potatoes a good toss. Pop the potatoes into the oven and roast for 20-25 minutes or until crispy and cooked through.

3. Heat a griddle pan over a high heat on the hob. Rub the remaining olive oil over the turkey burgers and carefully add them to the griddle pan. Cook the burgers for 2-3 minutes on each side before placing into the oven for 5 minutes. Once the burgers are cooked allow them to rest for 5 minutes.

4. Slice the ciabatta rolls in half and toast them. Spread with mayonnaise. Lay one tomato slice on the bottom half of each roll, followed by a turkey burger, and top with the other piece of bread. Serve with the potato wedges.

PER SERVING

CARBS	ENERGY	FAT	SATURATES	PROTEIN	SUGAR	FIBRE	SALT
79g	797 kcal	28g	5g	52g	15g	12g	1.25g

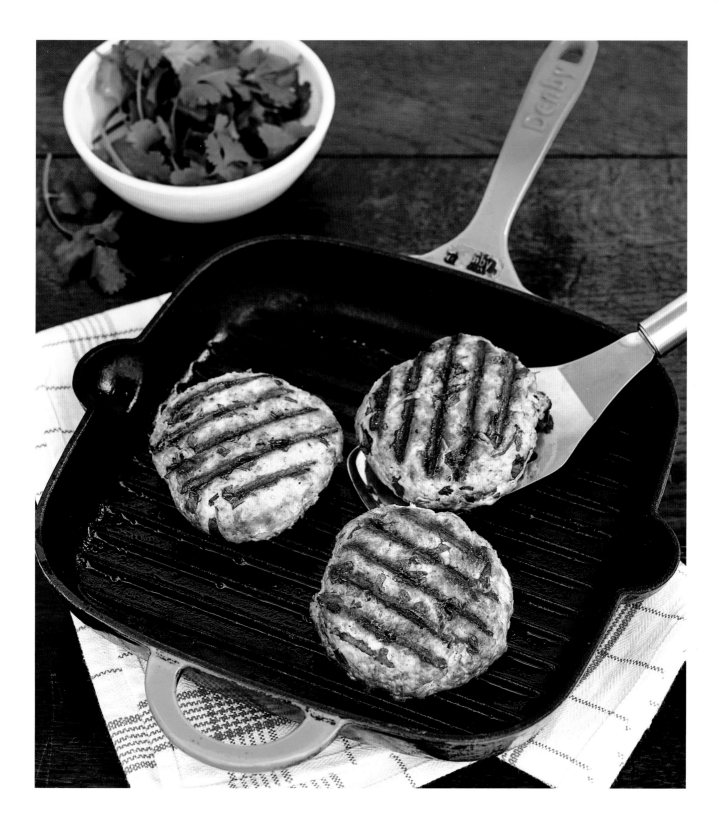

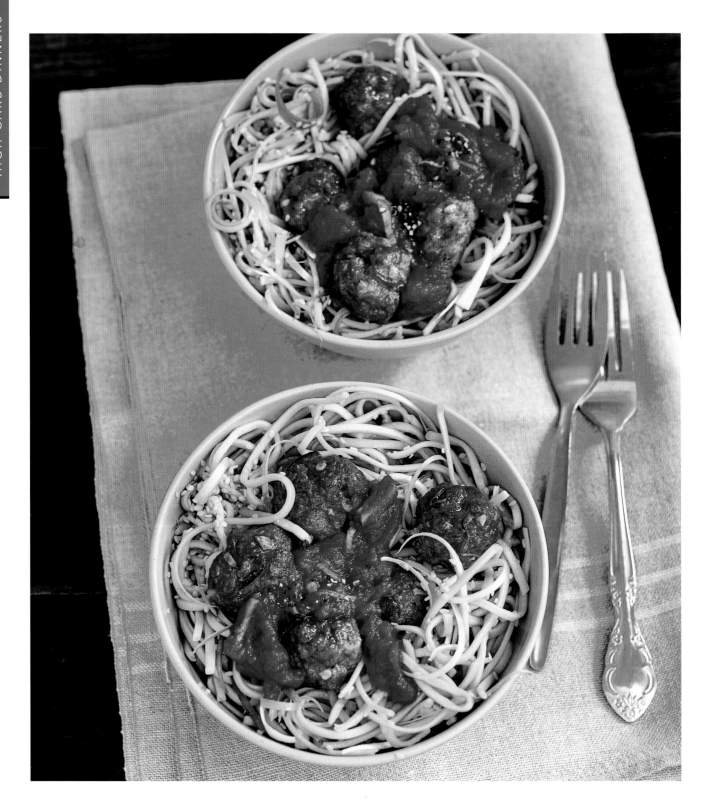

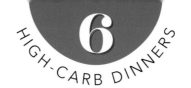
SWEET & SOUR PORK BALLS WITH SESAME NOODLES

SERVES **2** ◆ PREP TIME **15 MINS** ◆ COOK TIME **40 MINS** ◆ DIFFICULTY **EASY** ◆ **DF**

INGREDIENTS

350g pork mince
2 garlic cloves, finely sliced
1 red chilli, finely sliced

SWEET AND SOUR SAUCE
1cm piece ginger, finely sliced
400g tin chopped tomatoes
1 tablespoon soy sauce
1 tablespoon honey
150ml water
1 tablespoon white wine vinegar

SESAME NOODLES
150g dried egg noodles
1 tablespoon sesame oil
1 tablespoon sesame seeds
3 spring onions, finely sliced

METHOD

1. Preheat your oven to 180°C.

2. Place the pork mince in a large bowl. Add the garlic and chilli to the pork, season with salt and pepper and form into small balls (about the size of a 50p piece). Chill the pork balls in the fridge for 30 minutes. Then place them on a roasting tray and pop in the oven for 20 minutes.

3. Meanwhile, place all the ingredients for the sweet and sour sauce into a large saucepan and place over a high heat. Bring to the boil then turn down to a gentle simmer. Cook the sauce for 10 minutes. Now add the pork balls to the sauce and continue to simmer until needed.

4. Place the egg noodles in a large bowl and cover with boiling water from the kettle. Leave the noodles for 10 minutes to soften, then drain and place in a bowl. Now heat a wok over a high heat and add the sesame oil. Carefully add the noodles and toss well. Cook for 2-3 minutes then add the sesame seeds and spring onions. Toss well before dividing the noodles between 2 serving bowls. Top with the pork balls and sauce and serve.

PER SERVING

CARBS	ENERGY	FAT	SATURATES	PROTEIN	SUGAR	FIBRE	SALT
69g	737 kcal	29g	8g	48g	18g	6.5g	2.3g

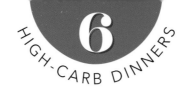

MAPLE & BALSAMIC ROASTED CHICKEN WITH POTATO & BEAN HASH

SERVES **2** ◆ PREP TIME **15 MINS** ◆ COOK TIME **30 MINS** ◆ DIFFICULTY **EASY** ◆ **GF** ◆ **DF**

INGREDIENTS

2 chicken breasts, skinless and boneless
2 tablespoons maple syrup
2 tablespoons balsamic vinegar
3 sprigs thyme, chopped
3 garlic cloves, finely chopped
1 bunch coriander, roughly chopped

POTATO HASH

1 large sweet potato, peeled and cut into 2cm dice
2 garlic cloves, finely chopped
400g tin kidney beans, drained
1 pinch ground cumin
1 pinch ground cinnamon
1 teaspoon smoked paprika
1 tablespoon olive oil

METHOD

1. Preheat your oven to 200°C.

2. First make the potato hash. Place the sweet potato chunks on a roasting tray and sprinkle over the chopped garlic. Now add the kidney beans to the tray and season with salt, pepper, cumin, cinnamon and paprika. Drizzle over the olive oil and give it a good mix. Pop some foil over the tray and roast the potato in the oven for 30 minutes or until cooked through.

3. Meanwhile, place the chicken breasts on another roasting tray and season with salt and pepper. Drizzle over the maple syrup and balsamic vinegar. Sprinkle over the thyme and garlic and place in the oven. Bake the chicken for 15 minutes or until cooked through. Now take a spoon and baste the sticky sauce in the bottom of the roasting tray over the chicken.

4. Remove the potato from the oven and divide between 2 plates. Top the potato with the chicken breasts and any sauce in the roasting tray. Sprinkle the coriander over the chicken and serve.

PER SERVING

CARBS	ENERGY	FAT	SATURATES	PROTEIN	SUGAR	FIBRE	SALT
60g	530 kcal	8g	1.5g	46g	23g	14g	0.4g

6 69014 44934 4

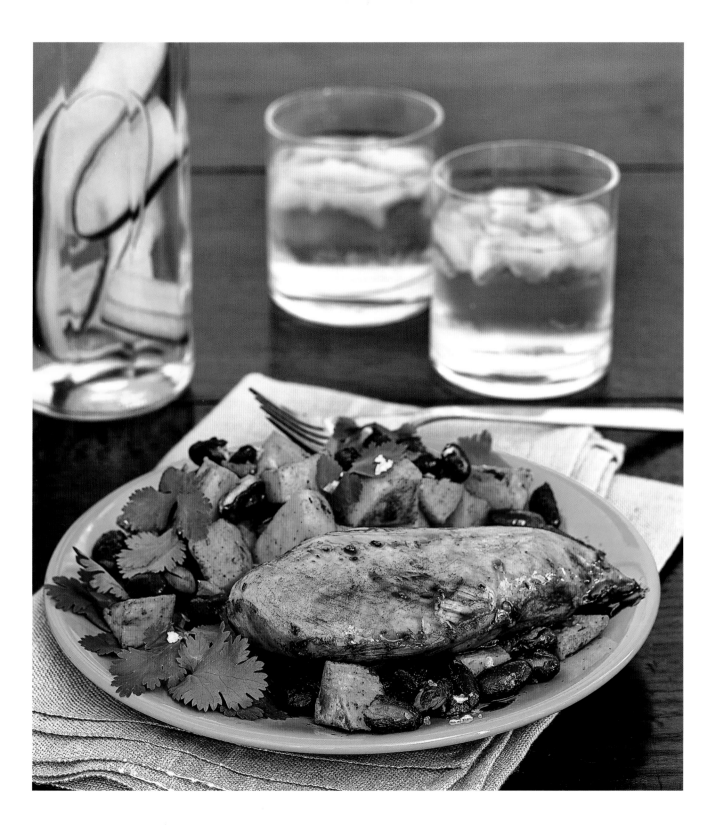

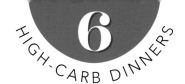

SPINACH, LEMON & BROAD BEAN RISOTTO

SERVES **2** ◆ PREP TIME **10 MINS** ◆ COOK TIME **45 MINS** ◆ DIFFICULTY **MODERATE**

INGREDIENTS
150g broad beans
1 tablespoon olive oil
2 garlic cloves, finely chopped
1 onion, diced
150g arborio rice
800ml chicken stock
2 handfuls baby spinach leaves
Zest and juice of 2 lemons
25g grated Parmesan cheese

OMAR SAYS: 'If all the stock is absorbed before the rice is cooked, add an extra ladleful of hot stock or water.'

METHOD
1. Half-fill a small saucepan with water and bring to the boil. Add the broad beans and cook for 2 minutes. Once the beans are cooked drain and run under cold water. Peel away the skins and set the beans aside.

2. Heat the olive oil in a medium-sized saucepan over a medium heat. Add the garlic and onion to the pan and cook for 2 minutes without colouring. Now add the rice to the pan and cook for a further 2 minutes, ensuring you keep the rice moving in the pan.

3. Carefully add a ladleful of the chicken stock to the pan and stir until all the liquid is absorbed and then add another ladleful of stock. Continue this process until the rice is cooked. Now fold in the baby spinach and broad beans. Season with salt and pepper and add the lemon zest and juice to the pan. Divide between 2 plates and serve with the Parmesan.

PER SERVING

CARBS	ENERGY	FAT	SATURATES	PROTEIN	SUGAR	FIBRE	SALT
73g	527 kcal	11.5g	4g	28g	7g	9g	0.9g

6 69014 44935 1

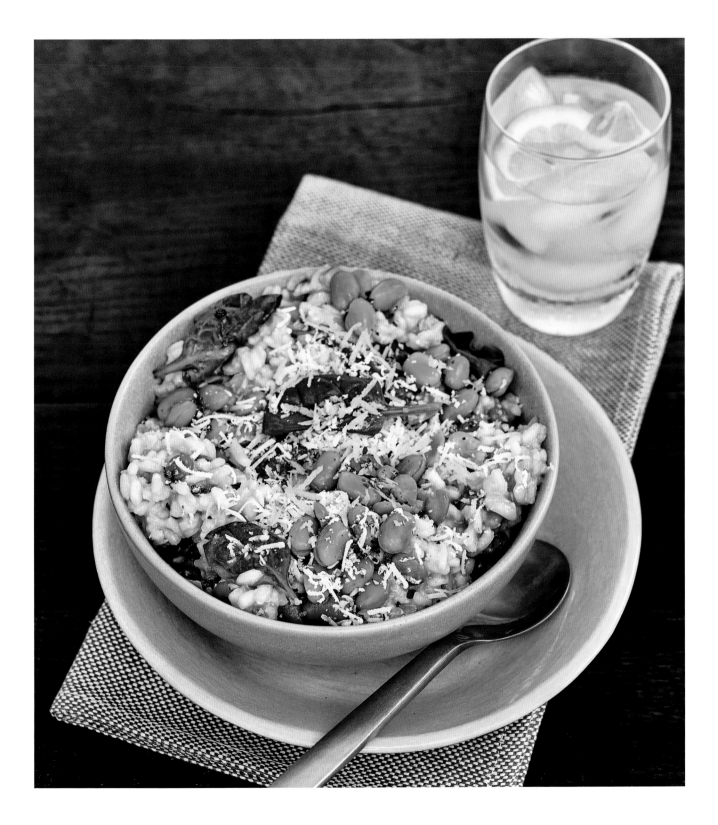

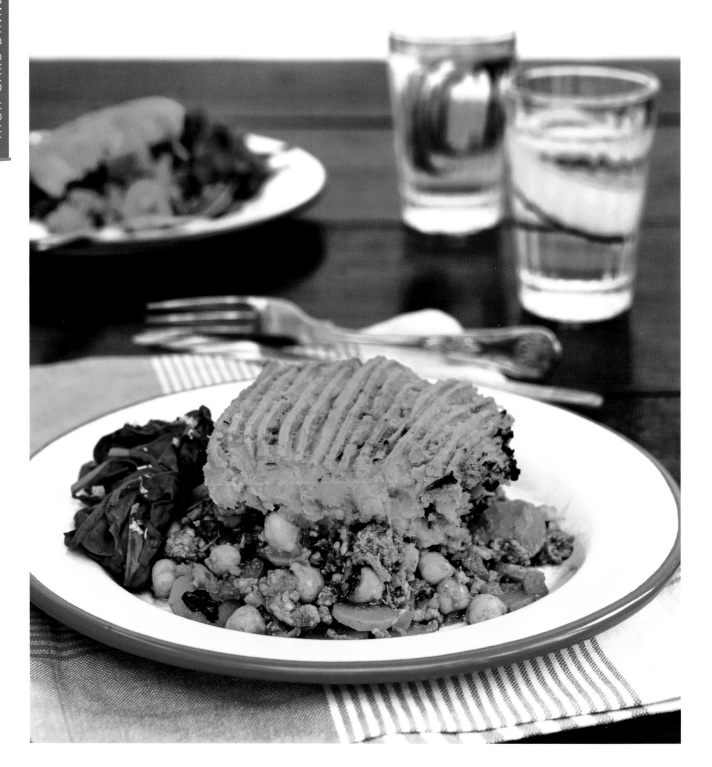

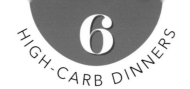

MOROCCAN SHEPHERD'S PIE WITH SWEET POTATO

SERVES **4** ◆ PREP TIME **10 MINS** ◆ COOK TIME **1 HR 25 MINS** ◆ DIFFICULTY **EASY** ◆ **GF** ◆ **DF**

INGREDIENTS

3 large sweet potatoes
1 tablespoon olive oil
1 onion, finely chopped
1 stick celery, finely chopped
2 garlic cloves, finely chopped
½cm piece ginger, finely chopped
1 carrot, peeled and finely chopped
400g lean lamb mince
1 teaspoon ground cinnamon
1 teaspoon ground cumin
1 teaspoon dried chilli flakes
1 tablespoon Meridian Yeast Extract
400g tin chopped tomatoes
150ml water
400g tin chickpeas
1 small bunch coriander, roughly chopped
1 sprig rosemary, roughly chopped

METHOD

1. Preheat your oven to 200°C. Pop the sweet potatoes on a roasting tray and bake in the oven for 35 minutes or until cooked through. Split them down the centre and carefully peel away the skin. Place the potato in a bowl and mash it with a fork. Set aside.

2. Heat the olive oil in a large saucepan over a high heat. Add the onion, celery, garlic, ginger and carrot to the pan and cook for 2 minutes without colouring. Now add the lamb mince and continue to cook for 5 minutes or until the lamb is browned all over. Add the cinnamon, cumin and chilli flakes. Now add the yeast extract, chopped tomatoes, water and chickpeas and continue to cook for 15-20 minutes. Season with salt and pepper. Fold the coriander into the meat.

3. Pour the meat into a casserole dish or deep baking tray and carefully spoon over the sweet potato mash, ensuring the meat is covered with potato. Sprinkle the rosemary over the top. Pop the shepherd's pie in the oven and bake for 20 minutes or until the potato is crispy and golden on top.

PER SERVING

CARBS	ENERGY	FAT	SATURATES	PROTEIN	SUGAR	FIBRE	SALT
64g	538 kcal	15g	6g	29g	20g	13g	0.9g

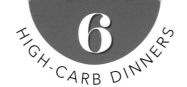

CHICKEN, DATE & CASHEW CURRY

SERVES **2** ◆ PREP TIME **5 MINS** ◆ COOK TIME **20 MINS** ◆ DIFFICULTY **EASY**

INGREDIENTS

2 chicken breasts, skinless and boneless
1 tablespoon olive oil
2 garlic cloves, finely chopped
½cm piece ginger, finely chopped
1 onion, finely chopped
2 tablespoons medium curry powder
½ teaspoon ground cinnamon
1 teaspoon ground turmeric
200ml (½ can) reduced-fat coconut milk
200ml water
2 tablespoons Meridian Date Syrup
3 tablespoons Meridian Cashew Butter
2 handfuls baby spinach leaves
4 spring onions, finely chopped
250g packet wholegrain steamed pilau rice

OMAR SAYS: 'The cashew butter gives the sauce a creamy texture.'

METHOD

1. Roughly chop the chicken breasts into 8 pieces and place in a bowl. Heat the olive oil in a large saucepan over a medium heat and add the garlic, ginger and onion and cook for 1-2 minutes without colouring. Now add the chicken and cook for a further 2 minutes. Add the curry powder, cinnamon and turmeric to the pan and cook for 1 minute.

2. Pour in the coconut milk, water, date syrup and cashew butter and bring to the boil. Turn the curry down to a gentle simmer and cook for 8-10 minutes, stirring occasionally. Add the spinach leaves and the spring onions and cook for 1 minute. Season the curry with salt and pepper.

3. Heat the pilau rice according to the packet instructions, divide between 2 plates and serve the curry alongside the rice.

PER SERVING

CARBS	ENERGY	FAT	SATURATES	PROTEIN	SUGAR	FIBRE	SALT
42g	662kcal	31g	11g	48g	17g	10g	0.75g

6 69014 44937 5

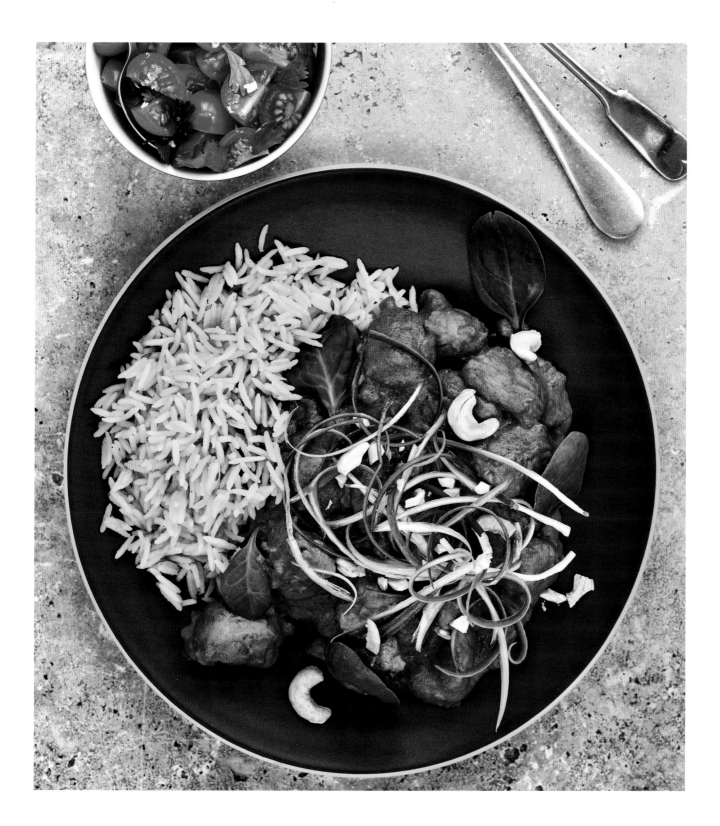

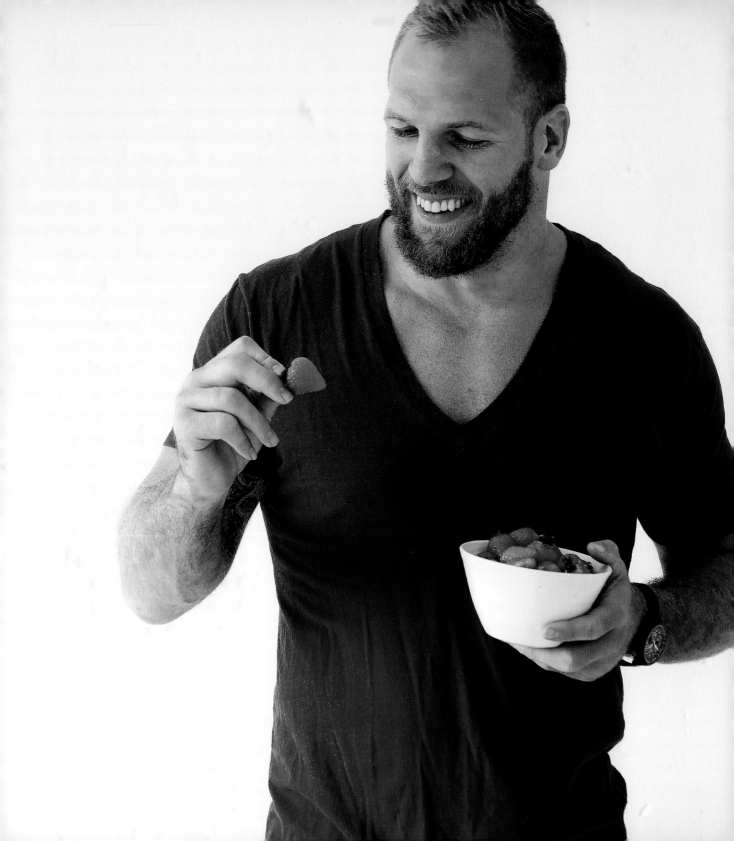

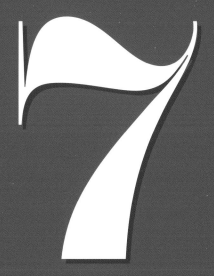

7

PRE-TRAINING SNACKS

You can be more relaxed about eating simple carbs pre-training, as your body will put them straight to good use as an immediate energy source.

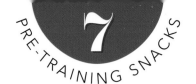

MIXED BERRY & GREEK YOGHURT SMOOTHIE

SERVES **2** ◆ PREP TIME **5 MINS** ◆ DIFFICULTY **VERY EASY** ◆ **V**

INGREDIENTS
100g blueberries
100g raspberries
100g strawberries
2 tablespoons oats
250g Greek yoghurt
250ml water

METHOD
1. Place all the ingredients in a food processor and blend until smooth and serve. Add a small banana if you prefer it a little sweeter.

PER SERVING

CARBS	ENERGY	FAT	SATURATES	PROTEIN	SUGAR	FIBRE	SALT
24g	278 kcal	14.5g	9g	10g	15g	6g	0.2g

6 69014 44938 2

BEETROOT & APPLE JUICE

SERVES **2** ◆ PREP TIME **10 MINS** ◆ DIFFICULTY **EASY** ◆ **GF** ◆ **DF** ◆ **VG**

INGREDIENTS
3 medium raw beetroots
1 green apple
3 medium carrots, peeled
½cm piece ginger

METHOD
1. Juice the beetroots first then the apple, followed by the carrots. Finely chop the ginger and add to the fresh juice.

PER SERVING

CARBS	ENERGY	FAT	SATURATES	PROTEIN	SUGAR	FIBRE	SALT
20g	113 kcal	1g	0.25g	2.5g	18.5g	2.5g	0.3g

6 69014 44939 9

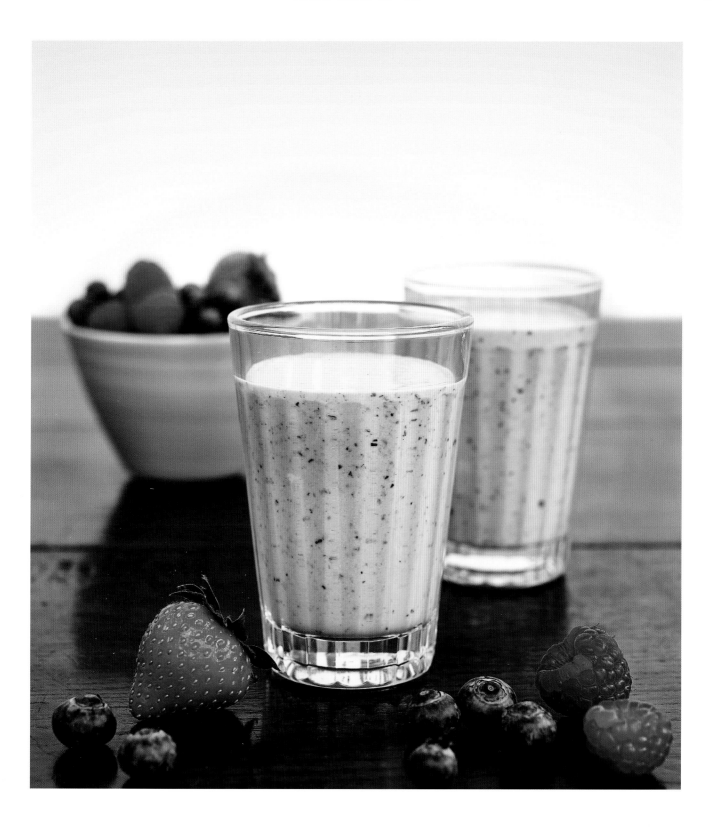

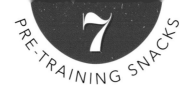

7

PRE-TRAINING SNACKS

BANANA & ALMOND SEEDY BARS

MAKES **8 BARS** ◆ PREP TIME **5 MINS** ◆ COOK TIME **30 MINS** ◆ DIFFICULTY **EASY** ◆ **DF** ◆ **V**

INGREDIENTS
3 ripe bananas
1 tablespoon coconut oil
3 tablespoons honey
2 tablespoons Meridian Almond Butter
1 teaspoon vanilla extract
300g oats
2 tablespoons ground linseeds
150g flaked almonds

METHOD
1. Preheat your oven to 180°C. Line a small baking tray with parchment.

2. Peel the bananas, place in a saucepan and mash until smooth. Add the coconut oil, honey, almond butter and vanilla extract to the saucepan and heat over a low heat. When the ingredients have melted together remove from the heat and pour into a large bowl.

3. Now add the remaining ingredients and give it a good mix. Pour the mixture into the lined baking tray and press down. Bake in the oven for 20 minutes or until golden brown.

4. Allow the tray to cool before cutting into 8 bars and serving.

PER SERVING

CARBS	ENERGY	FAT	SATURATES	PROTEIN	SUGAR	FIBRE	SALT
37g	368 kcal	18.5g	3g	11g	13g	5g	Trace

6 69014 44940 5

COTTAGE CHEESE, GRAPEFRUIT & MIXED BERRIES

SERVES **1** ◆ PREP TIME **5 MINS** ◆ DIFFICULTY **VERY EASY** ◆ **GF** ◆ **V**

INGREDIENTS
2 tablespoons cottage cheese
1 grapefruit, peeled
50g blueberries
50g strawberries, halved

METHOD
1. Place the cottage cheese in the bottom of a serving bowl. Segment the grapefruit and place on top of the cottage cheese. Place the blueberries and strawberries on top of the grapefruit and serve.

PER SERVING

CARBS	ENERGY	FAT	SATURATES	PROTEIN	SUGAR	FIBRE	SALT
18.5g	125 kcal	2g	1g	5g	18.5g	5.5g	0.2g

6 69014 44941 2

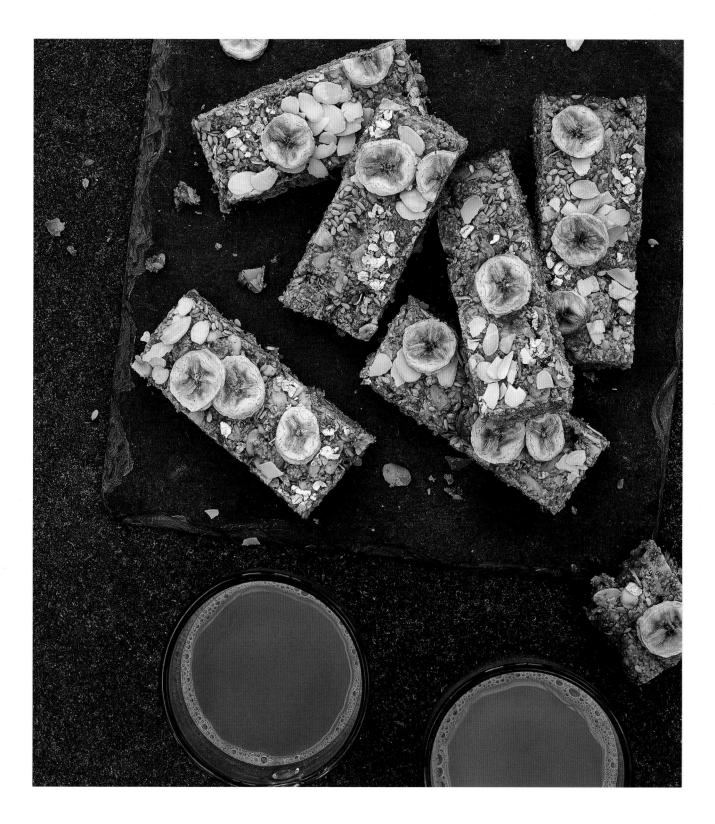

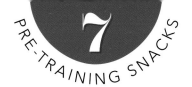

7

PRE-TRAINING SNACKS

MERIDIAN CHOCOLATE FLAPJACKS

MAKES **15** ◆ PREP TIME **5 MINS** ◆ COOK TIME **20 MINS** ◆ DIFFICULTY **EASY** ◆ **DF** ◆ **V**

INGREDIENTS

100g honey
100g Meridian Smooth Peanut Butter
400g oats
75g Meridian Cocoa & Hazelnut Butter

METHOD

1. Preheat your oven to 190°C and grease and line a 20cm square oven tin with baking paper. Mix together the honey, peanut butter and oats in a large bowl, then transfer the mixture to the prepared tin, pressing it down and into the corners with the back of a spoon to level the surface.

2. Bake for 20 minutes, until golden. Allow to cool slightly, and cut into 15 squares. Spread each square with a teaspoon of cocoa & hazelnut butter. Serve.

PER SERVING

CARBS	ENERGY	FAT	SATURATES	PROTEIN	SUGAR	FIBRE	SALT
25g	189 kcal	7g	1.5g	5g	8.5g	3g	Trace

FRUITY PROTEIN BARS

MAKES **16 BARS** ◆ PREP TIME **5 MINS** ◆ COOK TIME **5 MINS** ◆ DIFFICULTY **EASY** ◆ **VG**

INGREDIENTS

225g Meridian Almond Butter
115g maple syrup
330g oats
250g almonds
115g dried cranberries
115g pistachios
75g linseeds (or flax seeds)
75g walnut halves
85g sunflower seeds
115g pumpkin seeds
50g whey protein powder

METHOD

1. Line a small baking tray with parchment paper and set aside.

2. Pour the almond butter and maple syrup into a saucepan and place over a low heat. Warm until both have melted. In a mixing bowl combine all the remaining ingredients and mix well. Pour over the almond butter mixture and stir well.

3. Pour the mixture into the lined baking tray and press down firmly. Place the tray in the freezer for 1 hour. Remove from the freezer and cut into 16 bars and serve or place into an airtight container for later.

PER SERVING

CARBS	ENERGY	FAT	SATURATES	PROTEIN	SUGAR	FIBRE	SALT
26g	486 kcal	33g	3.5g	19g	10.5g	6g	Trace

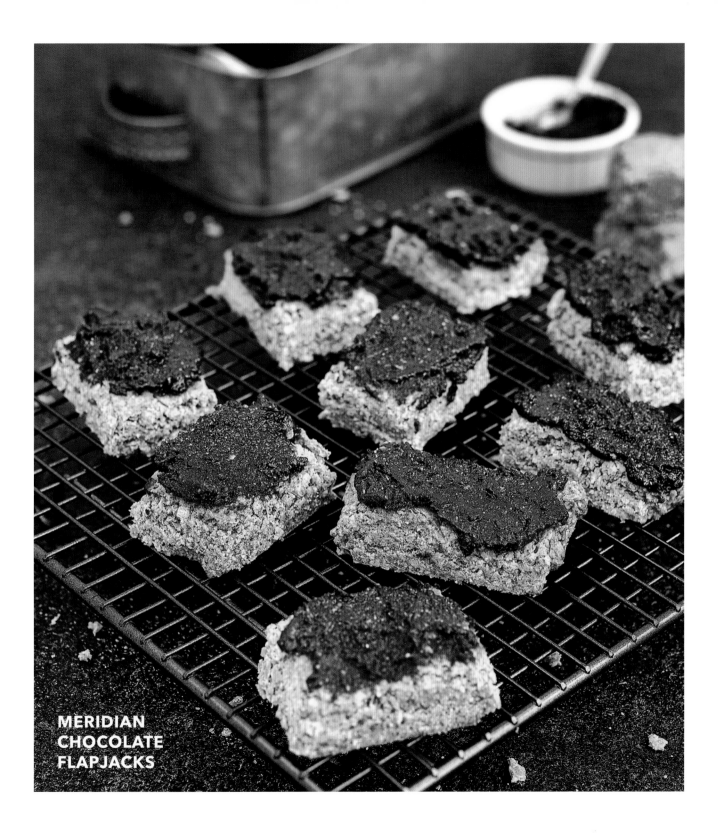

MERIDIAN
CHOCOLATE
FLAPJACKS

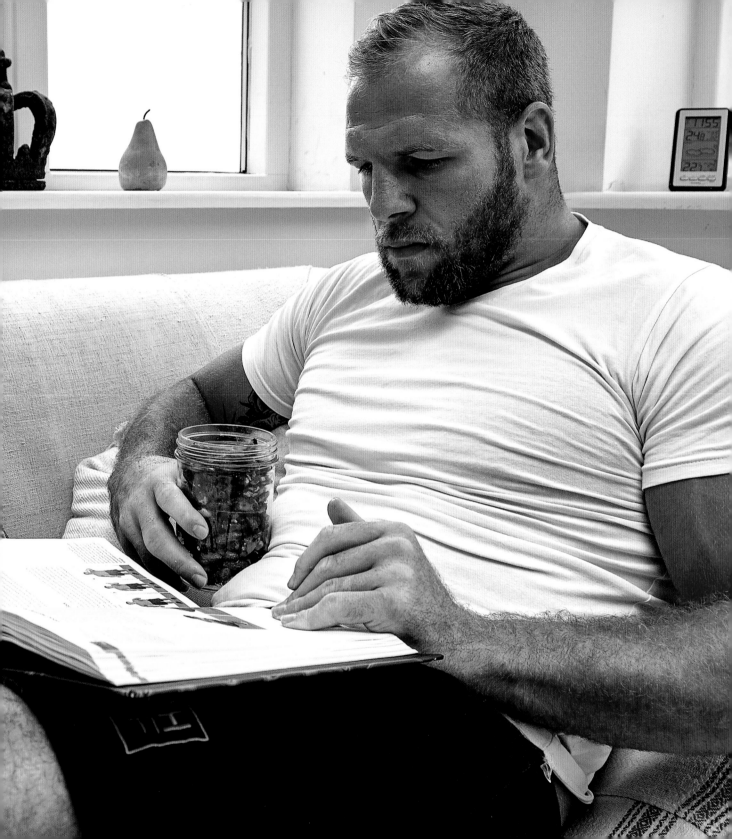

8

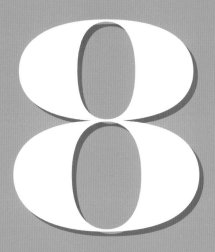

POST-TRAINING SNACKS

Eating healthy snacks after training or post-match can help with your recovery, as nutrients will be transported to your muscles quickly, encouraging rebuild.

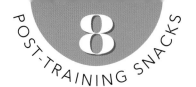

LEMON HUMMUS
WITH CRUDITES

SERVES **3-4** ◆ PREP TIME **10 MINS** ◆ DIFFICULTY **VERY EASY** ◆ **DF** ◆ **VG**

INGREDIENTS

400g tin chickpeas, drained
1 garlic clove
1 tablespoon Meridian Light Tahini
2 tablespoons olive oil
1 small bunch coriander
Juice of 1 lemon
1 carrot
½ cucumber
1 green apple

JAMES SAYS: 'The tahini adds protein, minerals and healthy fats. Serve with pitta bread for an extra energy boost.'

METHOD

1. Place the chickpeas, garlic, tahini, olive oil, coriander and a pinch of salt and pepper in a food processor and blend until smooth. Add the lemon juice to the hummus and stir. Transfer to a bowl.

2. Peel the carrot and cut into batons, then cut the cucumber into batons. Remove the core of the apple and cut into wedges. Serve with the hummus.

PER SERVING

CARBS	ENERGY	FAT	SATURATES	PROTEIN	SUGAR	FIBRE	SALT
19.5g	244 kcal	13.5g	2g	8g	7g	7g	0.1g

6 69014 44944 3

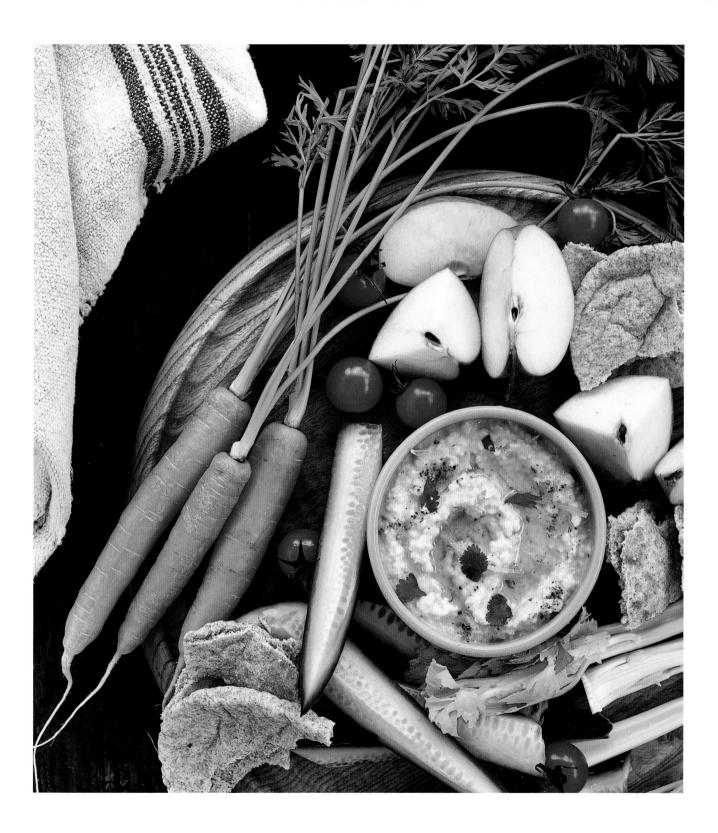

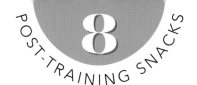

HONEY & CHILLI SPICED TRAIL MIX

MAKES **25 X 25G SERVINGS** ◆ COOK TIME **10 MINS** ◆ DIFFICULTY **EASY** ◆ **GF** ◆ **DF** ◆ **V**

INGREDIENTS
100g honey
1 teaspoon salt
½ teaspoon ground black pepper
½ teaspoon ground cumin
½ teaspoon ground coriander
½ teaspoon smoked paprika
1 pinch cayenne pepper
500g mixed nuts

METHOD
1. Preheat your oven to 200°C.

2. Mix all the ingredients together in a large bowl.

3. Pour the mixture into a roasting tray, ensure the tray is large enough to lay the nuts in one layer only. Roast in the oven for 8-10 minutes. Remove from the oven and allow to cool before transferring to an airtight container or Kilner jar.

PER SERVING

CARBS	ENERGY	FAT	SATURATES	PROTEIN	SUGAR	FIBRE	SALT
5g	131 kcal	10g	1.5g	5.5g	4g	0.5g	0.2g

6 69014 44945 0

CHERRY & COCOA SMOOTHIE

SERVES **2** ◆ PREP TIME **10 MINS** ◆ DIFFICULTY **VERY EASY** ◆ **GF** ◆ **V**

INGREDIENTS
175ml semi-skimmed milk
175ml water
250g pitted cherries
1 tablespoon cocoa powder
1 tablespoon ground almonds

METHOD
1. Place all the ingredients in a food processor and blend until smooth.

PER SERVING

CARBS	ENERGY	FAT	SATURATES	PROTEIN	SUGAR	FIBRE	SALT
19g	179 kcal	7.5g	2g	8g	18g	3g	0.1g

6 69014 44946 7

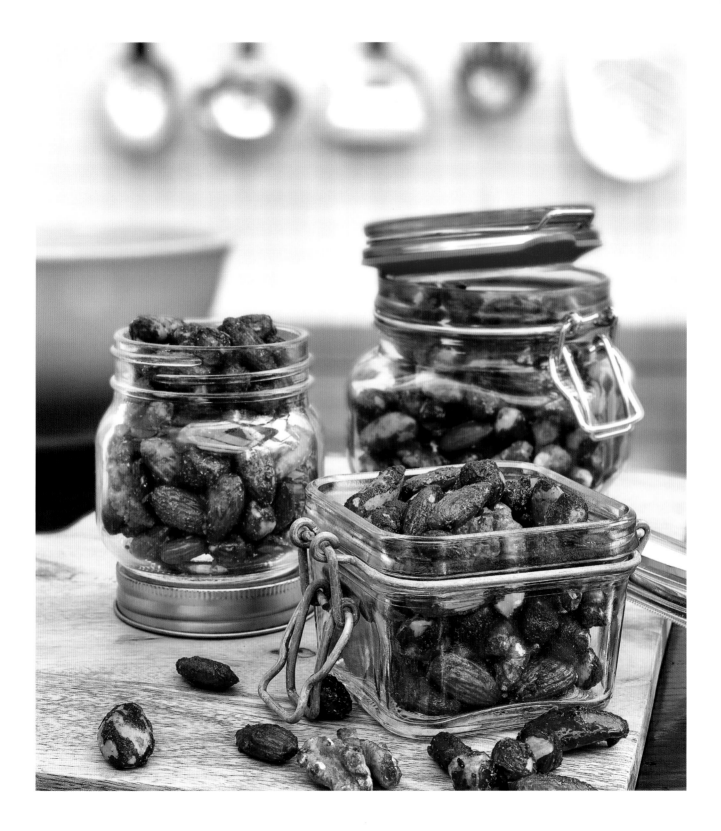

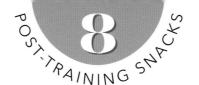

PEANUT BUTTER, COCOA & OAT BALLS

MAKES **12** ◆ PREP TIME **15 MINS** ◆ COOK TIME **5 MINS** ◆ DIFFICULTY **EASY** ◆ **DF** ◆ **V**

INGREDIENTS
85g honey
85g Meridian Peanut Butter
225g oats
2 tablespoons cocoa powder

METHOD
1. Pour the honey and peanut butter into a small saucepan and heat over a low heat. When the two have melted pour into a large mixing bowl. Now add the oats and cocoa powder and mix together. Form into approximately 12-15 balls and pop into the fridge for 10 minutes to firm up before serving.

PER SERVING

CARBS	ENERGY	FAT	SATURATES	PROTEIN	SUGAR	FIBRE	SALT
17.5g	142 kcal	5g	1g	5g	6g	3g	Trace

6 69014 44947 4

BOILED EGG, TOMATO & FIG SALAD

SERVES **1** ◆ PREP TIME **5 MINS** ◆ COOK TIME **5 MINS** ◆ DIFFICULTY **VERY EASY** ◆ **GF** ◆ **DF** ◆ **V**

INGREDIENTS
2 eggs
½ punnet cherry tomatoes, sliced in half
2 fresh figs, sliced

METHOD
1. Half-fill a small saucepan with water and bring to the boil over a high heat. Once the water is boiling add the eggs, bring to the boil again and time for 3 minutes. Remove the eggs and run under cold water. When the eggs have cooled peel away the shell and slice the eggs in half and place in a serving bowl.
2. Add the cherry tomatoes to the bowl with a pinch of salt. Serve the salad with the sliced figs alongside.

PER SERVING

CARBS	ENERGY	FAT	SATURATES	PROTEIN	SUGAR	FIBRE	SALT
11.5g	227 kcal	12g	3g	17.5g	11.5g	3g	0.9g

6 69014 44948 1

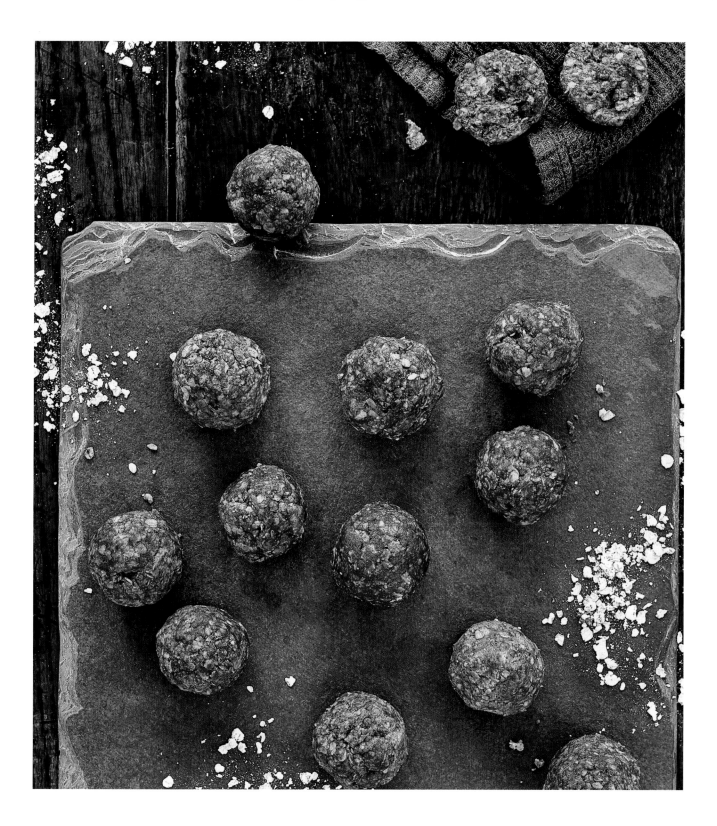

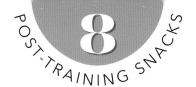

NUTTY COCOA BITES

SERVES **2** ◆ PREP TIME **5 MINS** ◆ DIFFICULTY **VERY EASY** ◆ **GF** ◆ **DF** ◆ **V**

INGREDIENTS
4 rice cakes, or 12 mini rice cakes
60g Meridian Cocoa &
Hazelnut Butter

METHOD
1. Spread 1 teaspoon of cocoa & hazelnut butter on each rice cake. Serve.

PER SERVING

CARBS	ENERGY	FAT	SATURATES	PROTEIN	SUGAR	FIBRE	SALT
13g	184 kcal	12.5g	2.9g	4g	2g	1.5g	Trace

6 69014 44949 8

TUNA SALAD WITH BOILED EGGS

SERVES **2** ◆ PREP TIME **10 MINS** ◆ COOK TIME **20 MINS** ◆ DIFFICULTY **EASY** ◆ **GF** ◆ **DF**

INGREDIENTS
4-5 new potatoes
50g edamame beans
50g French beans
2 eggs
2 tomatoes, quartered
1 spring onion, finely sliced
½ red onion, finely sliced
1 tablespoon olive oil
1 teaspoon white wine vinegar
½ baby gem lettuce
1 small tin tuna in spring water, drained

METHOD
1. Place the potatoes in a small saucepan and cover with water. Bring to the boil over a high heat. Cook for 10 minutes or until cooked through. Drain and run under cold water. Pat the potatoes dry and slice into halves.
2. Half-fill a small saucepan with water and bring to the boil. Add the edamame beans and bring the water back to the boil. Add the French beans. When the water is boiling again cook for 1 minute then drain and run under cold water. Pat the edamame beans dry and slice the French beans in half.
3. Half-fill a small saucepan with water and bring to the boil. Carefully place the eggs in the water. As soon as the water begins to boil again time for 3 minutes. Remove the eggs and run under cold water. Peel the shell away from the eggs and slice them in half.
4. Place the tomatoes, spring onion and red onion in a mixing bowl. Add the potatoes and beans. Drizzle over the olive oil and vinegar and toss well. Roughly chop the baby gem lettuce and place in the bottom of a serving bowl, then top with the salad. Spoon the tuna on top of the salad and serve.

PER SERVING

CARBS	ENERGY	FAT	SATURATES	PROTEIN	SUGAR	FIBRE	SALT
25g	328 kcal	13g	2.5g	25g	8.5g	6.5g	0.35g

6 69014 44950 4

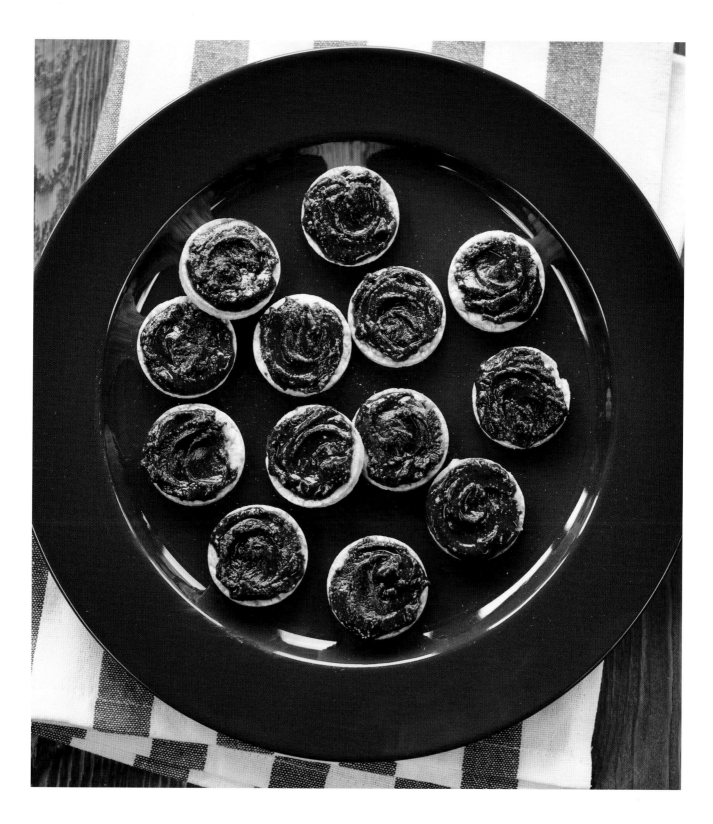

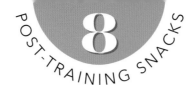

BANANA BREAD WITH PUMPKIN & SUNFLOWER SEEDS

SERVES **12** ◆ PREP TIME **10 MINS** ◆ COOK TIME **55 MINS** ◆ DIFFICULTY **EASY** ◆ **DF** ◆ **V**

INGREDIENTS

3 very ripe bananas
2 tablespoons Meridian Pumpkin Seed Butter
2 tablespoons Meridian Sunflower Seed Butter
100g caster sugar
1 teaspoon vanilla extract
1 teaspoon bicarbonate of soda
½ teaspoon baking powder
1 egg
200g plain flour
1 tablespoon pumpkin seeds
1 tablespoon sunflower seeds

JAMES SAYS: 'For a lower-carb version use a sugar substitute, eg Truvia.'

METHOD

1. Preheat your oven to 180°C.

2. Place the bananas in a large bowl and mash with a fork. Now add the pumpkin seed and sunflower seed butters and mix. Next add the sugar, vanilla, bicarbonate of soda, baking powder and egg and mix until combined. Fold in the flour.

3. Line a small loaf tin with baking parchment and pour in the banana bread mixture. Sprinkle the pumpkin seeds and sunflower seeds over the top and pop it into the oven. Bake for 50-55 minutes to 1 hour or until cooked through. Check with a skewer after 50 minutes. If it comes out clean it's done. Once the banana bread is cooked allow it to cool before slicing and serving.

PER SERVING

CARBS	ENERGY	FAT	SATURATES	PROTEIN	SUGAR	FIBRE	SALT
27.5g	168kcal	4g	0.6g	4.5g	13g	1.5g	0.3g

6 69014 44951 1

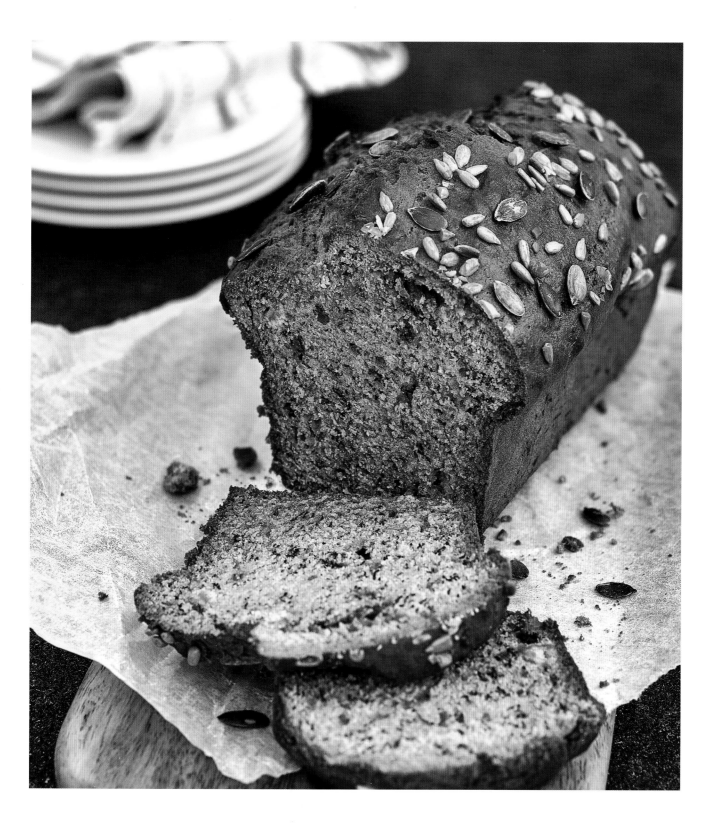

CONTRIBUTORS

EDITOR:
MARGARET NICHOLLS

Margaret is a London-based editor. Following 20 years as editor-in-chief of the lifestyle department at the UK's biggest magazine publisher, she is currently working as a freelance writer, editor and project manager. Specialities include food, health, lifestyle and real life.

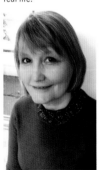

CREATIVE DIRECTOR:
GINO TAMBINI

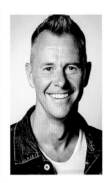

Gino Tambini has art directed or designed for most of the top-selling consumer magazines in the UK. He has shot front covers, fashion, lifestyle and food on location around the world. He now runs his own design company, working in London for the country's major publishers, and producing high-end book designs and branding projects from his studio in Surrey.

EDITOR-AT-LARGE:
JONATHAN HASKELL

Father of James and his official 'gofer' (second class), Jonathan started his career in the fashion business, moving into the world of corporate branding and merchandising. Finally, having sold his business, he ended up as Senior Vice President Europe, Middle East and Asia, for Michael C. Fina, the global Employee Reward and Recognition company.

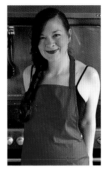

FOOD STYLIST:
LIZ O'KEEFE

Former chef, food stylist, food writer and recipe developer, Liz O'Keefe is home economist on LandScape magazine, producing British seasonal recipes for each issue, and food stylist for many large commercial clients, as well as cookery books. Liz has published two of her own books, *The Great British Pepper Cookbook* and *The Mushroom Cookbook*.

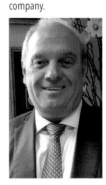

FOOD PHOTOGRAPHER:
CLIVE BOZZARD-HILL

Having studied architecture, Clive moved into the world of photography in the mid 1980's. Working across various genres, he has specialised in food photography for the past 20 years. Clive enjoys skiing, diving and would love to learn to fly!

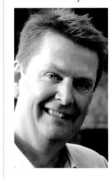

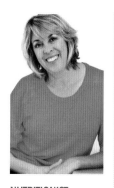

NUTRITIONIST:
FIONA HUNTER

After graduating with a degree in nutrition and post-graduate diploma in dietetics, Fiona worked as a dietitian in the NHS, before joining *Good Housekeeping* magazine. Now freelance, she works with the media, publishers and the food industry.

FOOD ASSISTANT:
HELEN RANCE

Primarily based in London, Helen has been styling for over 15 years. With experience across media, advertising, packaging and retail, she has worked with many established household brands, leading super-markets and high street institutions.

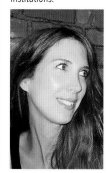

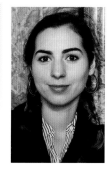

PROP STYLIST & FOOD ASSISTANT:
HANNAH SEARLE

Hannah is a prop stylist and food stylist assistant living and working in London. She specializes in sourcing and styling props for food and lifestyle photography and has worked extensively with brands such as Tesco, Sainsbury's and Boots.

PROOFREADER-IN-CHIEF:
SUSIE HASKELL

Mother of James and the only sane one in the family! Aside from being ace at all things spelling and grammar, Susie runs her own very successful corporate gifts and promotional merchandising business, and boasts a glittering array of household name companies on her client list. Her claim is that she can personalise anything!

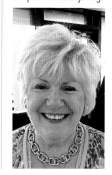

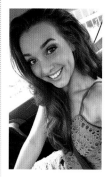

FILMING CO-ORDINATOR:
HANNAH MITCHELL

Hannah has recently graduated with a 1st class honours degree in Fashion and Textiles and has extensive experience in coordinating both photo and film shoots. She has worked on a variety of projects within music and fashion before specialising in the fitness and food industry.

SPECIAL THANKS TO...

As with most things in life, when we embark on a new project we think we know what we are doing, only to be rapidly confronted by the reality that actually we don't have the faintest idea!

This is what happened to me with *Cooking for Fitness*. I knew in headline terms exactly what I wanted to achieve and impart. I feel so passionately about exercise and training that my previous books have focused primarily on these areas. But with this book I wanted to shine a light on the equally important area of food.

I knew exactly what I wanted to achieve: a cookery book full of fitness-friendly recipes that were easy to prepare but still incredibly tasty.

And I wanted to show that cooking from scratch using fresh ingredients does not have to be complicated or difficult.

However, unlike a work of fiction, where you just need an author, a sheet of paper and a pen, I soon discovered that creating a cookery book requires an entirely different level of complexity... and a team of experts with very specific skills.

Naturally, the first person I turned to was my old friend **Omar Meziane,** who back in the day was the executive chef at Wasps before he moved on to stratospheric heights with the multiple gold medal winning GB Olympic Rowing Squad and then to fantastic success with the Men's England Football Team, where he cooked them into the semi-finals of the 2018 World Cup.

The brief to Omar was concise: to create a range of simple recipes which even someone new to cooking could readily master. They had to be nutritious, delicious but above all quick and easy to make. As ever, Omar delivered... and how!

So there we were with the recipes all sorted, ready to be cooked and photographed. That's when the realisation hit. How exactly do we bring all this to life?

Luckily, help was at hand. A lovely lady called **Charlotte Jones** kindly gave me the name of exactly the right person: the inspirational cookery expert and food stylist **Liz O'Keefe.**

To our great fortune, Liz was between projects and said she could help.

'This is what we need,' said Liz, rattling off a list of things that had never remotely occurred to me. *Studio set, props, prop specialist, food photographer, food stylist...* and so the list went on.

That's when I first met the photography legend that is **Clive Bozzard-Hill** and **Helen Rance,** the prop queen.

So off Omar and I went to the studio and two weeks later, with Liz's stellar help on the food styling front, we had cooked and shot all 79 recipes. Brilliant, I thought, that's it.

'No, no, no,' said Liz. 'That's just the start! You

> *Creating a cookery book requires a team of experts with very specific skills*

need a top nutritionist to go through every recipe with a fine toothcomb, and to analyse all the quantities and ingredients. Then you need a first rate designer to reflect all the superb photography and showcase the recipes in a way that makes them compelling as well as easy to follow.

'Lastly, you need a brilliant editor to join the whole lot together and bring the book to life.'

'I know just the people,' said Liz, and she was totally right.

First, nutritionist **Fiona Hunter** demonstrated her forensic knowledge of every ingredient and was a real star.

Next, creative director **Gino Tambini** proved that he is a truly great and innovative designer, and absolutely nailed it.

Finally, our wonderful editor **Margaret Nicholls** kept a steady but firm hand on the tiller, making sure the whole production process moved seamlessly along to a brilliant conclusion.

But the honours don't end there…

Huge thanks must go to my old man **Jonathan,** who as publisher and editor-at-large oversaw the entire production and creative process from start to finish and who has worked tirelessly to bring the whole project to fruition. And to my mother **Susie,** for once again grasping the mantle of all the proofreading as well as bustling around in the background doing all the unseen bits.

In addition to our chief photographer Clive,

I can't thank these people enough. It truly has been a great collaboration

credit must go to the rest of our film and photography team: cameraman **Barry Curran,** who filmed all the brilliant videos of Omar and me cooking away; **Neil Cooper** for the great front cover images as well as other portraits of Omar and myself;

Hannah Mitchell, the filming co-ordinator, who was thrown in at the deep end but came up smelling of roses; and **Helen Searle,** who worked alongside Liz on phase two of filming.

Printing plaudits go to our production team of **Tugba** and **Kubra,** as well as **Baris,** the main man at our printer's and a real source of support.

My gratitude to **Sue** and **Darren** from Meridian Foods, as well as **Sue** and **Nas** from Promote PR for their unstinting support and assistance with this project.

Lastly, but by no means least, my amazing and lovely girlfriend **Chloe,** who kept me well fed and watered on Omar's brilliant recipes and, when I faltered, picked me right back up again and gave me the motivation to see it all through to the end.

I can't thank all of these people enough. They are a skilled and hard-working group without whom none of this could have happened. It truly has been a great collaboration.

I really hope you have enjoyed reading *Cooking for Fitness* and that you get as much fun and pleasure out of cooking the recipes as Omar and I had in creating them.

YOUR INSTANT NUTRITION TRACKER

KEEP YOUR FITNESS GOALS ON TRACK WITH OUR HANDY RECIPE BARCODES – THEY LINK DIRECTLY TO THE MYFITNESSPAL APP…

If, like me, you track your nutrition using the MyFitnessPal app – or you would like to start doing so – then this recipe book will make it a whole lot easier for you!

To save you time and effort, we have created a barcode for every recipe and linked it with the MyFitnessPal app so that you can instantly scan it without having to input it manually.

As on the recipes themselves, the nutritional values are worked out per portion.

HERE'S HOW THE APP WORKS:

♦ Whether your goal is weight loss or weight gain, the MyFitnessPal app recommends a daily calorie intake calculated to help you achieve your target.

♦ Every day, you simply log your food intake and exercise into the app's diaries. MyFitnessPal will calculate how many calories and/or macros you need to consume for the rest of the day.

♦ The app contains thousands of foods in its database, including fresh produce like fruit and vegetables as well as many branded and supermarket products, plus meals and drinks in restaurants.

♦ The app can also scan barcodes on food packaging and automatically logs the nutrition information on your diary.

USING THE APP WITH THIS BOOK:

♦ Every recipe in *Cooking for Fitness* comes with a barcode linked to the app. Simply scan the barcode and the app will instantly show the recipe's nutritional values and add them to your food diary. You can find the barcodes on the recipe pages as well as on our handy index starting on page 197.

♦ If you're using a computer instead of a phone, or the barcode scanner won't play ball, log in to the app, go to 'Add Food' and type 'James Haskell plus the recipe name' in the search box, eg: 'JAMES HASKELL BAKED EGGS WITH KALE, SPINACH & PARMESAN', and the nutritional values will appear. Alternatively, type in the barcode number, and that will work too.

♦ Just a note about salt: the values in the app are given as sodium rather than salt, but they are correct. 1g salt = 400mg sodium.

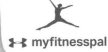

1
LOW-CARB BREAKFASTS

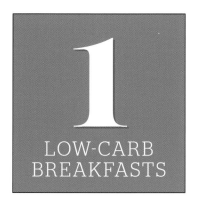

PAGE 40 BAKED EGGS WITH KALE, SPINACH & PARMESAN

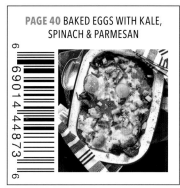

PAGE 42 BEETROOT & MACKEREL FRITTATA

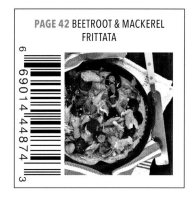

PAGE 44 SMOKED TROUT WITH AVOCA-DO & COTTAGE CHEESE WITH SEEDS

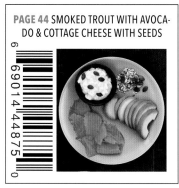

PAGE 47 SPICY OAXACA SCRAMBLED EGGS WITH SPINACH

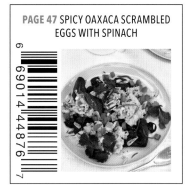

PAGE 48 DARK CHOCOLATE, PECAN, ALMOND & HONEY YOGHURT POT

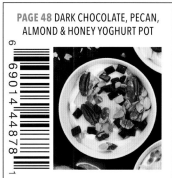

PAGE 48 MANGO, PASSION FRUIT & LIME YOGHURT POT

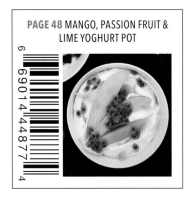

PAGE 51 MIXED BERRIES, HONEY & GRANOLA YOGHURT POT

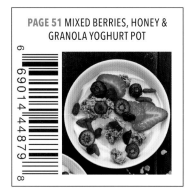

PAGE 51 CHERRY & ALMOND YOGHURT POT

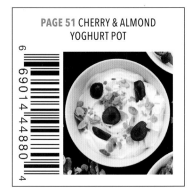

PAGE 52 AVOCADO, HAM & CHILLI TARTS

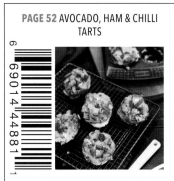

PAGE 55 BACON, JALAPENO & BUTTER BEAN OMELETTE

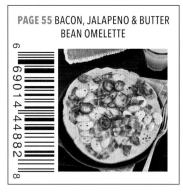

PAGE 56 HOMEMADE SAUSAGES, EGGS & AVOCADO

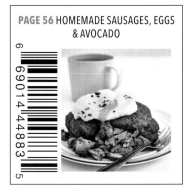

PAGE 58 SUPER GREENS SMOOTHIE

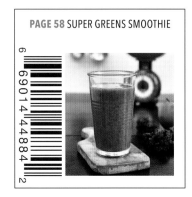

2
HIGH-CARB
BREAKFASTS

PAGE 62 BANANA & PEANUT BUTTER FRENCH TOAST

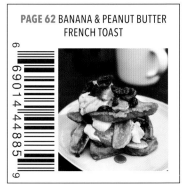

PAGE 64 SWEET POTATO, BUTTER BEAN & AVOCADO HASH

PAGE 67 JAMES'S FULL ENGLISH BREAKFAST

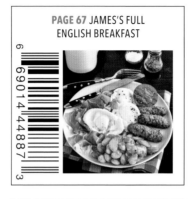

PAGE 68 MEXICAN CHORIZO BREAKFAST BURRITO

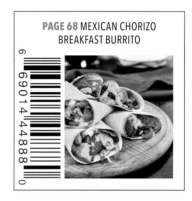

PAGE 70 BREAKFAST BRUSCHETTA

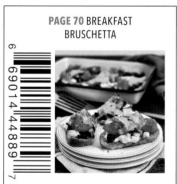

PAGE 73 SPINACH, POTATO & CHILLI FRITTERS WITH BOILED EGGS

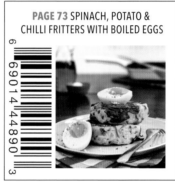

PAGE 74 EGGS ROYALE WITH YOGHURT HOLLANDAISE

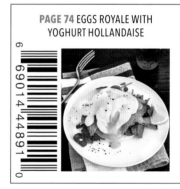

PAGE 76 BIRCHER MUESLI

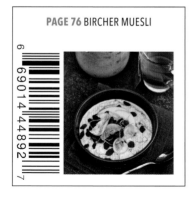

PAGE 79 HOMEMADE BEEF SAUSAGE SANDWICH

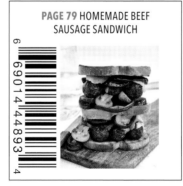

PAGE 80 LEFT-OVER CHICKEN KEDGEREE

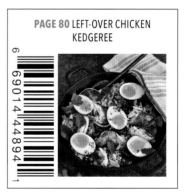

PAGE 82 PASSION FRUIT, COCONUT & ALMOND CHIA

PAGE 82 PEANUT BUTTER & BANANA CHIA

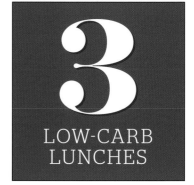

3
LOW-CARB LUNCHES

PAGE 86 TRICOLORE SALAD

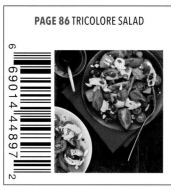

PAGE 88 SPINACH, GINGER & CHILLI BALLS WITH THAI MANGO SALAD

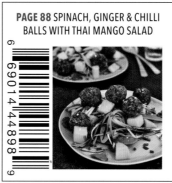

PAGE 91 SPICY SQUID WITH BLOODY MARY TOMATO SALAD

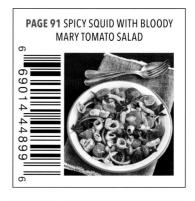

PAGE 92 TURKEY WITH BEETROOT & STILTON SALAD

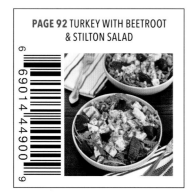

PAGE 92 MACKEREL WITH SWEET CHILLI SAUCE

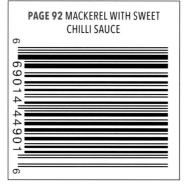

PAGE 94 CHICKEN SHAWARMA SALAD BOWL

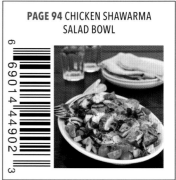

PAGE 96 TOMATO & BUTTER BEAN
SOUP WITH ROASTED COD

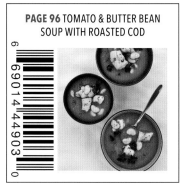

PAGE 98 CURRIED CHICKEN &
ROASTED CAULIFLOWER SALAD

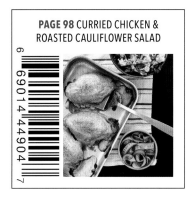

PAGE 101 SKINNY LIME & CORIANDER
PORK BURGER WITH CRUNCHY VEG SALAD

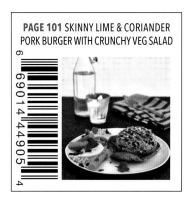

PAGE 102 PRAWN LAKSA

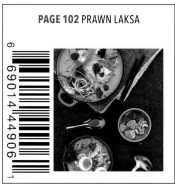

PAGE 104 SMOKED SALMON
FLATBREAD PIZZA

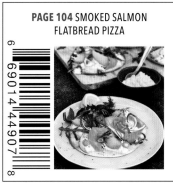

4

HIGH-CARB
LUNCHES

PAGE 108 RAINBOW SALAD WITH
SPICY RICE & TURKEY

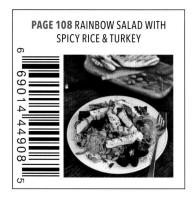

PAGE 110 SPICY MEXICAN BEEF
QUESADILLAS

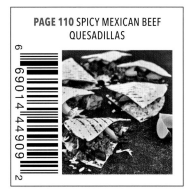

PAGE 113 SWEET POTATO, CHICKPEA &
KALE SOUP

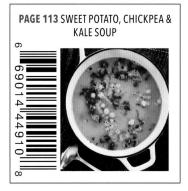

PAGE 114 POSH MACKEREL
FISH FINGER SANDWICHES

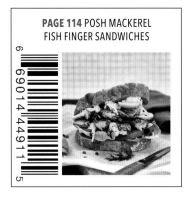

PAGE 116 TURKEY, CHORIZO & PAPRIKA
MEATBALLS WITH CHILLI POTATO SALAD

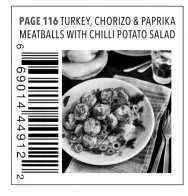

PAGE 119 TABBOULEH SALAD WITH
ROASTED SALMON

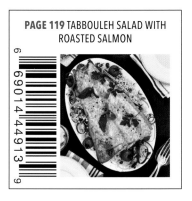

PAGE 120 LAMB KEBABS WITH SPICY
RICE & APPLE SLAW

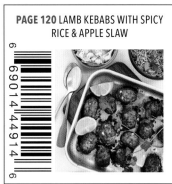

PAGE 122 QUINOA, SWEET POTATO &
BEETROOT SALAD WITH FETA

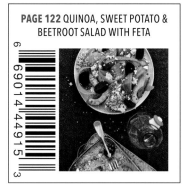

PAGE 125 CHICKEN GYROS WITH
LEMON POTATOES

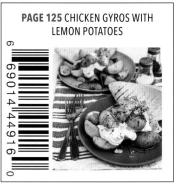

5
LOW-CARB
DINNERS

PAGE 128 FILLET STEAK WITH PARSNIP
MASH & WATERCRESS

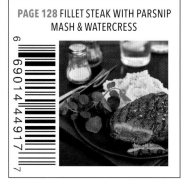

PAGE 130 JAMES'S LOW-CARB
SUNDAY ROAST

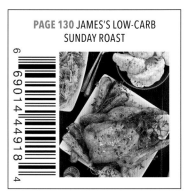

PAGE 133 SATAY CHICKEN WITH PAPAYA & CHILLI SALAD

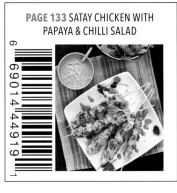

PAGE 134 COURGETTE BEEF LASAGNE

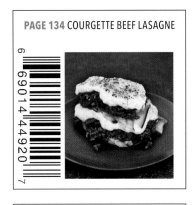

PAGE 137 TERIYAKI-GLAZED TUNA WITH STIR-FRIED PAK CHOI

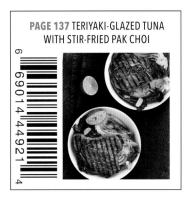

PAGE 138 BEAN FALAFEL WITH KALETTE & APPLE SALAD

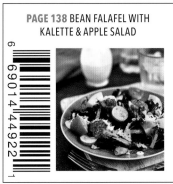

PAGE 140 CURRIED PORK CHOP WITH INDIAN CUCUMBER SALAD

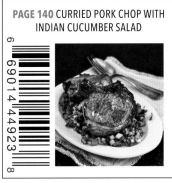

PAGE 143 PESTO & FETA FRITTATA WITH ROASTED BROCCOLI SALAD

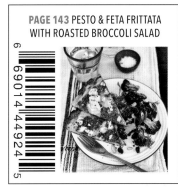

PAGE 144 LAMB CHOPS WITH ROASTED VEGETABLES & SALSA VERDE

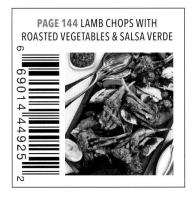

PAGE 146 ROASTED DUCK WITH MOLASSES & AUBERGINE SALAD

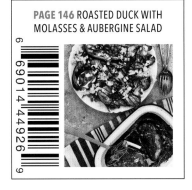

6
HIGH-CARB DINNERS

PAGE 150 JAMES'S FISH & CHIPS

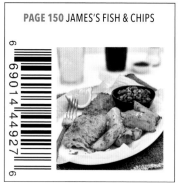

PAGE 152 SEA BASS WITH GINGER & TAMARI, BOILED RICE & EDAMAME BEANS

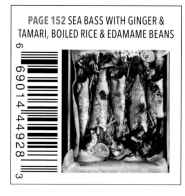

PAGE 155 PERI-PERI CHICKEN FEAST

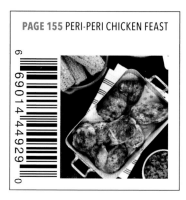

PAGE 156 JAMES'S FISH PIE

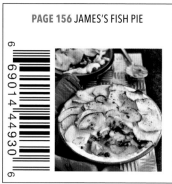

PAGE 158 MASSAMAN BEEF CURRY

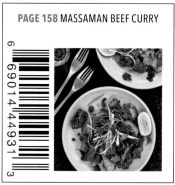

PAGE 160 CURRIED TURKEY BURGER WITH SWEET POTATO WEDGES

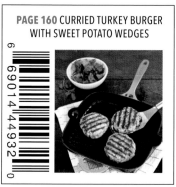

PAGE 163 SWEET & SOUR PORK BALLS WITH SESAME NOODLES

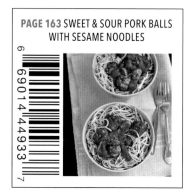

PAGE 164 MAPLE & BALSAMIC ROASTED CHICKEN WITH POTATO & BEAN HASH

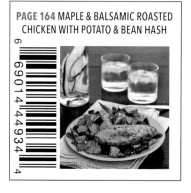

PAGE 166 SPINACH, LEMON & BROAD BEAN RISOTTO

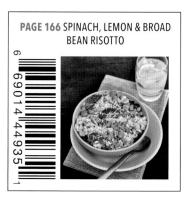

PAGE 169 MOROCCAN SHEPHERD'S PIE WITH SWEET POTATO

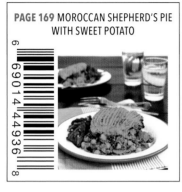

6 69014 44936 8

PAGE 170 CHICKEN, DATE & CASHEW CURRY

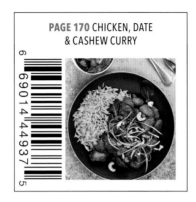

6 69014 44937 5

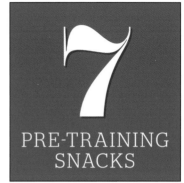

7

PRE-TRAINING SNACKS

PAGE 174 MIXED BERRY & GREEK YOGHURT SMOOTHIE

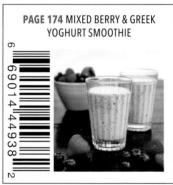

6 69014 44938 2

PAGE 174 BEETROOT & APPLE JUICE

6 69014 44939 9

PAGE 176 BANANA & ALMOND SEEDY BARS

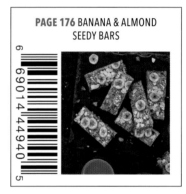

6 69014 44940 5

PAGE 176 COTTAGE CHEESE, GRAPEFRUIT & MIXED BERRIES

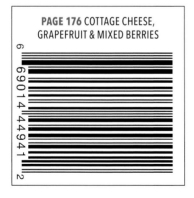

6 69014 44941 2

PAGE 178 MERIDIAN CHOCOLATE FLAPJACKS

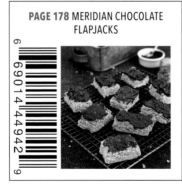

6 69014 44942 9

PAGE 178 FRUITY PROTEIN BARS

6 69014 44943 6

8
POST-TRAINING SNACKS

PAGE 182 LEMON HUMMUS WITH CRUDITES

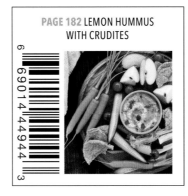

PAGE 184 HONEY & CHILLI SPICED TRAIL MIX

PAGE 184 CHERRY & COCOA SMOOTHIE

PAGE 186 PEANUT BUTTER, COCOA & OAT BALLS

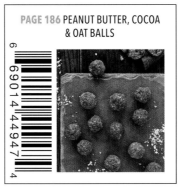

PAGE 186 BOILED EGG, TOMATO & FIG SALAD

PAGE 188 NUTTY COCOA BITES

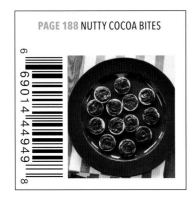

PAGE 188 TUNA SALAD WITH BOILED EGGS

PAGE 190 BANANA BREAD WITH PUMPKIN & SUNFLOWER SEEDS

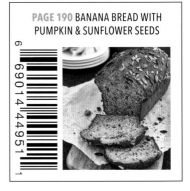

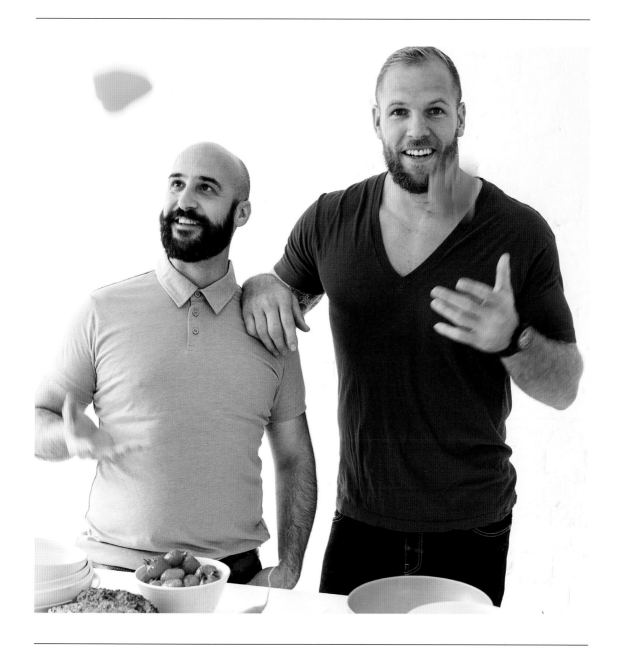

INDEX OF INGREDIENTS
& RECIPES

ABOUT THE AUTHORS...

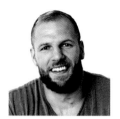

JAMES HASKELL

JAMES HASKELL, British & Irish Lion, Wasps, and now Northampton Saints, is one of the UK's most famous current rugby internationals, with over 78 England caps to date. He is equally well known for his impressive physique and dedicated attitude towards training and fitness.

James is highly respected for his comprehensive knowledge of fitness and nutrition, garnered from years of working with the country's top training and sports nutrition experts. His fans and followers on social media seek his advice on a daily basis on how best to eat and train.

And James is on a mission to share this knowledge. Both his body transformation book *Perfect Fit* and his rugby training guide *Rugby Fit* were bestsellers.

James knows from personal experience that 75 per cent of any successful exercise plan hinges on a good diet. And that it's equally important for recipes to be easy to prepare and delicious. That's why, with *Cooking for Fitness,* he turned to his friend and favourite chef Omar Meziane.

"I have never felt this fit or strong in my life"

Phil Robins, The Times (after following James's six-week programme in Perfect Fit)

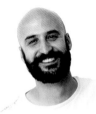

OMAR MEZIANE

OMAR MEZIANE is one of the UK's top performance chefs. Currently Executive Chef to the Men's England Football Team, he was a vital member of the behind-the-scenes team who helped propel the players to the semi-finals of the 2018 World Cup in Russia.

Previously chef to the GB Olympic Rowing Squad and Wasps rugby team, Omar is a master at devising menus for the country's elite sportsmen and women to help them perform at their peak.

Omar believes strongly that food should be healthy, but that it also has to be delicious. His cooking style is loosely based around his Mediterranean heritage, using plenty of herbs and spices to make it as flavoursome as possible.

Omar has appeared in the Hairy Bikers Home Comforts series for the BBC, as well as Channel 4's Food Chain. He also helped develop the award-winning National Lottery's Food Champion's website, giving an insight into the daily menus of athletes from across Team GB.

"Omar is the UK's top performance chef, he totally transformed the squad and we've never looked back"

Danny Welbeck, England and Arsenal

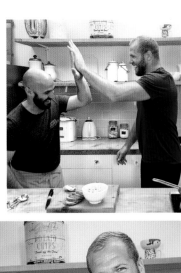

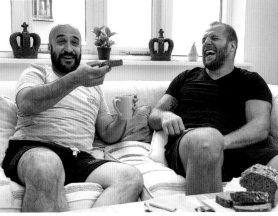

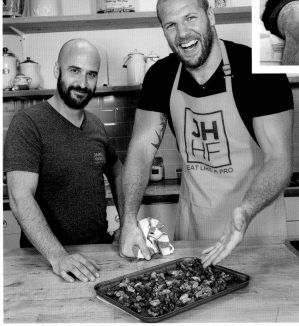

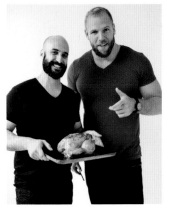

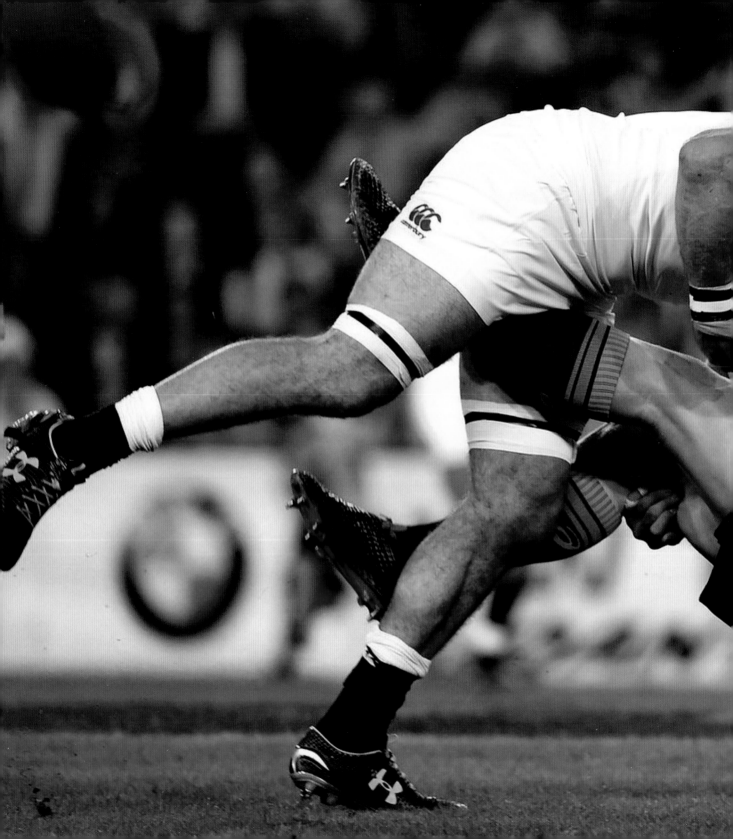

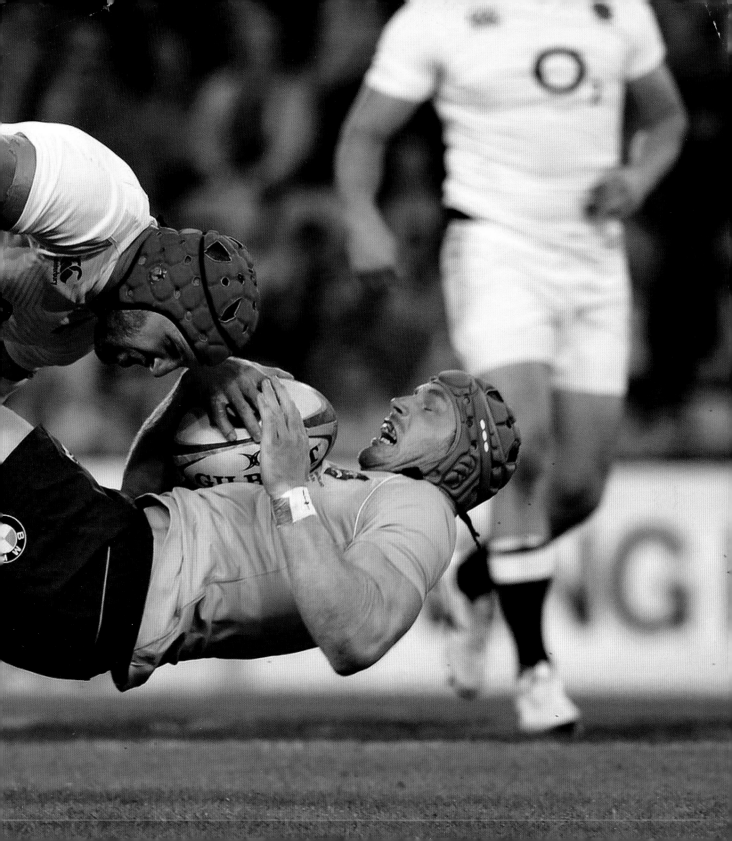

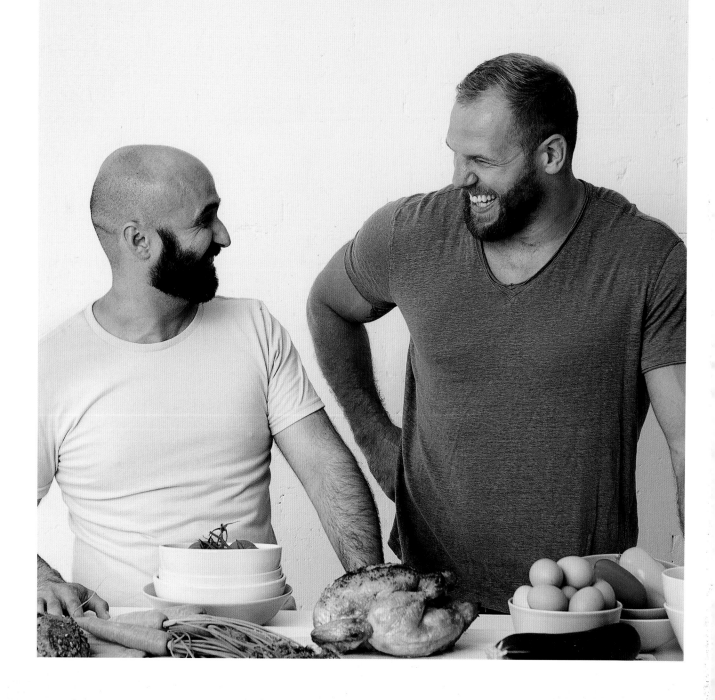

FITNESS STARTS IN THE KITCHEN